# THE CANCER IDOL

*A journey of hope and healing for ordinary believers
facing the monster.*

## By Frederick Tamagi

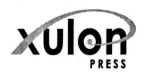

# ACKNOWLEDGMENTS

I would first like to thank my friend Hope, whose conversation with God over seven years ago became my first spiritual confirmation and the title for this book. I would also like to thank Dr. Sandra Kennedy (Whole Life Ministries - Augusta, Georgia, U.S.A.) for her foundational teaching of the Word that helped open the door to the rest of my life. With my utmost love, I would like to thank the small, private circle of family and friends that walked beside me, prayed with me, hoped with me, and most importantly, believed with me. You know who you are. Most of all, I give my worship and praise to Jesus Christ my Healer, to the Holy Spirit my Teacher, and to Almighty God, Who **is** the rest of my life.

# TABLE OF CONTENTS AND SCRIPTURE REFERENCES

# INTRODUCTION

This book is not meant to be a blueprint for healing. It isn't one of those wholly confident, thinly veiled, "name it and claim it" manuals about "God's Guaranteed Healing Provision for You!" As detailed and as literary as it may be, this book is, at its core, a story of an experience. It is a story about a very ordinary person, a very ordinary Christian believer, who was abruptly and brutally confronted with the extraordinary reality of cancer.

It is a story about fear. It is about experiencing a depth of fear that, if we are not believers, can easily overwhelm our natural lives, and if we are believers, might also influence our eternal destiny in the bargain.

It is a story about searching. Not the contented, peaceful searching conducted inside a Wednesday night Bible study or a quiet, secluded monastery. It is about searching, with not-so-quiet desperation, for a saving, healing Truth that is more real than earthly reality.

It is a story about wonder, as well — unexpected, inexpressible wonder. Picture this ordinary person, having very ordinary, even below-average expectations of God, experiencing His wonder, today, as if living in spiritual companionship with other "ordinary" citizens of Scripture like Gideon, Elijah, and Isaiah.

It is a story about a conversation. The conversation began with a desperate cry from a stricken child, and was answered, almost spontaneously, by a merciful voice emanating from the Word of God. This voice spoke from deep inside the Scriptures, out of the mist of dreams (sleeping and waking), from the pages of books and media, from the lips of anointed friends and family. There were times when this dialogue virtually took place in real time, with active, living responses to real questions. There were times when this dialogue took place in that contemplative, prayerful, "secret place" where most believers are taught that such exchanges might occur. This dialogue was offered in many different forms. It was clear that God's inexplicable grace followed me wherever I went, to whatever height or depth or circumstance I stumbled or bumbled toward.

It is a story about power. Often, we are subject to the power that can best influence us, satisfy us, frighten us, tranquilize us, and even destroy us. This may be the truth about power in this world. In our "enlightened" quest for this truth, we have been deceived; some willingly, some unwittingly. Many of us have surrendered to the power that we believe is a ruler and destroyer without peer. Having surrendered, we are frightened and intimidated into blindness and idolatry; and then, we are destroyed. So, we long for the power that is a Healer and a Savior without peer. We wonder if we will find Him.

Most of all, this story is about a Word. It is about a Word that is not just the pious title that we have given to a revered, ancient book of wisdom. It is about a Word that lives, breathes, thinks, and actually speaks to us. This Word is spoken from the heart, mind, and mouth of this Savior without peer. And, it is a personal Word, spoken with love and power, intended for an ordinary person. The Savior wants that person to be you.

I'm not sure who will eventually read this book. I would imagine that constituency to be anyone from schoolboy to scholar, invalid to valedictorian, fisherman to physician. With that in mind, I'll ask that you read this book in the light of the following qualifications.

1. I am, decidedly, not a Biblical scholar, nor a student of theology. I do hold a university degree, but my apprehension of Scripture and related material is founded solely on my very ordinary, "spiritual everyman" response to such matters. My approach to reading the Bible was not based on any organized or sanctioned study methodology, but rather on a methodology prompted by longing, desperation, and a broken heart. I suspect that this will be criticized by "serious" Bible scholars, professional or not, but my experience has made me wonder: How are God's "words" best received? Through the system or through the spirit? In any event, this question will remain unresolved, since my entire book was "received" and written via this very unscholarly medium of understanding.

2. In a related topic, those same serious Bible folks will probably notice that I am using a lot of "theologically incorrect" terms for impressions and images that I received on this journey. For example, I have used terms like "demon," "spirit," "idol," "stronghold," and "empire" to identify the underlying, evil agent and infrastructure of cancer in our world. I know that there is probably a literal difference between a demon and an evil spirit, or a stronghold and an empire, but I hope that the reader will not get "hung up" on the detail, but instead will see the larger panorama of God's story. The use of these terms, and others, occurred quite spontaneously as I received and recorded my impressions throughout the experience (which continues to this day). I apologize for the seeming inconsistency in my use of terms, but I have

tried to remain faithful to the images and words that God gave me at the time of writing.

3. A few months ago, I sent a couple of sample chapters of my manuscript to a Christian book editor. Although I received a positive response to my writing content, style, and expression, such was not the response to my alleged theology, based on this very limited submission. In view of that critique, I need to state, "up front" as it were, that:

- I do not believe that cancer is the only disease with an evil or demonic foundation. There are many other "incurable" and lethal diseases such as ALS (Lou Gehrig's Disease), Multiple Sclerosis, AIDS, etc., that may well originate from a similar evil source. Admittedly, I do speak of the unique nature of cancer, especially from the perspective of the massive earthly institution it has spawned, which is almost church-like in its trappings. However, I have written about cancer mainly because I had cancer and was given "light" concerning its spiritual underpinnings.

- I do not think that God's decision to withhold healing (or heal in His own way) is a personal failure of faith to be laid at the feet of the stricken believer. The view that adequacy of personal faith is the sole linchpin connecting us to divine healing has become a twisted source of condemnation (and exclusion) for thousands of ordinary, afflicted believers. The question of healing is far more complex and too supernatural to be left solely to the normal, precarious state of human faith. Exposing this cruel misconception, that we must first possess great personal faith to receive healing, is actually a crucial element in bringing more "ordinary" believers to a healing opportunity. Faith is a gift that God wants to give to everyone. A gift is most greatly prized by one who does not possess it, authentically desires to have it, and who cannot possibly obtain such a gift through self-effort. What disheartens many an afflicted believer is the perceived absence of this intended gift of faith. It may well have been "dispatched" by the healing will of God, but has simply not arrived yet. The post office can trace a personal, registered letter that has been sent, but is currently somewhere inside the system. It is my hope that more afflicted believers will search for this personal faith "letter" inside His Word, the Bible. I wrote this reply to the book editor when she accused me of equating death from illness with inadequate faith: "If great faith was a prerequisite for being healed, I should not have survived."

4. Throughout the book you will notice comments about the medical community involved in the treatment of cancer: doctors, nurses, technicians, caregivers. On many occasions I refer to them in a purely practical or earthly context, and on still other occasions I discuss them in the context of the spiritual. I have tried to be accurate and careful as I write in either context. However, you might be provoked by frequent references to this community as "priests of the idol," unwitting "temple dwellers," or even involuntary participants in the "delusion of the enemy" that permeates the cancer establishment. These references are part of the spiritual understanding that God gave me as I engaged the medical community who faithfully battle this incredible disease. In order to rebut any argument that I believe this community is somehow

active or complicit in the spiritual evil of cancer, I need to make the following points:

- I do not think that cancer doctors, nurses, technicians, or caregivers are demon-possessed, idol worshippers, or in any way acting as willing agents of the enemy.
- I do think they are (for the most part) skilled, compassionate, committed individuals who are dedicated to fighting a horrible, earthly disease.
- I do think they care deeply for cancer victims and their families.
- I do think these same caring individuals are both soldiers and victims in a battle that goes far beyond the purely clinical.
- I do think this caring community functions, diligently, inside an earthly institution that they are challenged to manage and control. Yet, at the same time, they are unwilling functionaries in the spiritual battle that rages within the institution.
- I do think many members of the cancer care community believe that their fight is much more than medical.

To the readers of this experience, I can only say that everything you will read actually happened. I will admit to only commencing the journey on my own. On the other hand, I guess you could argue that God started me on this journey when He allowed the illness in the first place. This, of course, would not have been my first choice. Regardless of how you may resolve that technical point, once I responded to the cancer diagnosis with a cry to God, He took over the rest of the trip.

I'm not sure how the travelogue ended up being so detailed and long. As you read, you may get angry, energized, puzzled, frightened, or even bored. Some of the chapters contain extensive, multiple images from Scripture. I can't really apologize for any reaction you may have because of the book's length or detail. Though the story is about me, the words are not mine. I'm trusting that the Holy Spirit will inspire you to "hang in there" as the story unfolds. I believe that it will be well worth your while.

If you are reading this story because you have cancer, no matter what kind of believer you think you are, no matter what portion of my story you accept or don't; this is my hope and prayer:

- That you will seek the will of God for your life with all of your heart.
- That you will seek His will, prayerfully and desperately, inside the words of Scripture.
- That through the mystery of Scripture and His other provisions, you will discover that God's will is a healing will.
- That your heart will receive news of your healing as a personal message from Him to you, spoken from deep inside His Word.

Most of all, I pray that this story will help you turn away from the great cancer idol and toward the great cancer Healer. May you worship no other gods before Him. May He speak to you. May you hear Him. May His Word be true. Amen.

# CHAPTER 1

# IT BEGINS

October 7,2002: An examination in my family doctor's office to evaluate small lumps on the right side of my neck, just above my collarbone. They had just appeared within the last week or so, and combined with the existing larger lumps under and in back of my right-side jaw, I was beginning to believe that I had more than just a routine dental infection.

For eight months previous, starting with a major dental procedure (bone graft) on that same side of my mouth, I had been trying to get a diagnosis (and treatment) for a small, swollen lymph node under the right side of my jaw. The lump had appeared, coincidentally, after the bone graft was done. My dentist had speculated that it was just a sympathetic lymph node reaction to the trauma caused by the recent procedure. He prescribed antibiotics and, for the next several weeks (and checkups) he seemed unconcerned and confident that it would eventually right itself. Finally, in March 2002, I went to my family doctor and asked for his evaluation. He was a little suspicious about the size and texture of the node, but after hearing the dental background, decided to put me on a stronger, extended regimen of antibiotics to reduce, and hopefully eliminate, the lymph node. A month later I returned to his office, and the lymph node had reduced a little, so he decided to take a "wait and see" attitude. The dental explanation still seemed the most plausible.

During this same period of time, I was also seeing a homeopathic doctor who had been of great help for a chronic, digestive problem I had been fighting. He had prescribed various homeopathic remedies to boost my immune system and, hopefully, reduce the lymph node. The next couple of months passed with no real visible change in the node, and then my homeopath suggested that I undergo special "testing." It was an electronic, acupuncture point, stimuli-response system. Through this test we would determine the cause of the enlarged lymph node. I submitted to the testing, and, remarkably, the test yielded a diagnosis of deep infection in the gum/jawbone area. Needless to say, I was relieved to finally have a reasonable idea as to what was causing my problems, and I was referred to another dentist who specialized in treating this type of infection. The first examination confirmed the suspicion of the homeopath. An x-ray showed an infection in the jawbone area adjacent to my most troubled, root-canalled, porcelain-crowned tooth. The dental specialist recommended extraction of the tooth, combined with deep cleaning of the socket, to be followed with a strong antibiotic. This procedure would alleviate the lymph node problem. In September 2002, I had my tooth extracted, and I confidently took the antibiotics which would finally solve the problem. A couple of weeks passed, and still the lymph node remained enlarged. The dentist felt that, since the extraction socket was still healing, the lymph node was "a continuing reaction to local trauma." Over the next week, the second set of swollen lymph nodes appeared quite suddenly above my collarbone, and I returned to my general practitioner.

This October examination, in my family doctor's office, was really the beginning of an incredible, multi-layered journey; clinically and emotionally human to the core, but, at its very center, deeply spiritual. As I look back upon that moment, I realize that my doctor's reaction, as he felt the second set of lymph nodes, became a strange kind of foreshadowing. His normally friendly, reserved facial expression was suddenly transformed into a visibly disturbed, even frightened appearance. His voice trembled as he murmured, "Oh no, Oh hell, Oh no..." His use of the word "hell" was quite uncharacteristic for this very kind doctor, and it wasn't until later that I realized that the reference indicated a kind of deep, irrational horror. It was a horror that most people feel when confronted with the world I was about to enter into. After a moment had passed, he told me that he definitely suspected "something pathological" now as opposed to infectious, because "these lymph nodes above the collarbone almost never enlarge due to infection." My response was to the point: "You mean cancer," I said, and he nodded yes. I was in quiet shock. Because of the pattern of lymph node enlargement and the absence of other obvious indicators, he speculated that it might be a lymphoma cancer, "which in most cases, is very treatable and curable." "One of the best kinds of cancer to get" (do you believe that?). I don't know if I was relieved or just less terrified, but it brought some calm to the situation. We were both in shock. At the same time, I know that we both wondered how the last 8 months of investigation could have been so misleading, so confusing, so damaging. "I wish I had reacted in April when I last saw you." (Yeah, me too, doc...) "We need to get you a chest x-ray and biopsy right away." And so it began.

I should mention that for many weeks prior to this moment, I was spending a lot of time on the computer researching my symptoms on the Internet. It was my first exposure to the virtually unlimited pool of medical information available. Right from the beginning of the journey in February, I was anxious for the answer to my situation.

Now, after the suspicion of cancer had been spoken, I spent the next few days intensively researching my specific symptoms. Just as my doctor had said, the initial appearance and pattern of the lymph nodes suggested lymphoma; hopefully Hodgkin's lymphoma, which was considered the most treatable. In cases of early detection, Hodgkin's was "eighty to ninety percent curable" (my first encounter with the dark statistics of cancer). It was a "wake-up call," to be sure, but perhaps a situation still under control.

About a week later, Lori and I found ourselves sitting in the doctor's office to discuss the results of the chest x-ray and needle-aspiration biopsy. He regretfully informed us that, while the chest x-ray was clear (indicating that no other lymph nodes, nor my lungs, were affected), the biopsy had indicated that the enlarged lymph nodes were not a result of lymphoma. It was, instead, a "squamous cell carcinoma of occult origin, probably in the head or neck region." This meant that there was a primary tumor somewhere else in my body that had already spread (metastasized) to the lymph glands on my neck. He sounded very serious as he stated that, "we **hate** this type of cancer," almost as if it were some sort of evil personage. We sat in quiet shock. He didn't want to comment much more. He said that he could only recall a handful of his patients, in his entire career, who had developed this type of cancer. So he couldn't really comment on prognosis, other than the fact that he was very, very sorry. He would refer me right away to a top head and neck specialist at the cancer clinic. Still more quiet shock, and oh yes, fear.

That very night, I spent hours on the Internet again, scanning the thousands of sites containing information about the new name that my "enemy" had been given ("squamous cell carcinoma of the head and neck"). The information was uniformly discouraging for a normally healthy person. I was used to seeing curable disease as a necessary "bump in the road" for some people, and incurable disease as an unfortunate, tragic experience for others. My mind and heart were bombarded by the endless statistics, studies, probabilities, and evidence of diminishing returns. These were the cold, hard facts about my cancer. By the time cancer moves to the lymph nodes, it's very serious, unpredictable, and often uncontrollable. The information gets progressively more bleak and foreboding as you understand more of what modern medicine is up against. I kept on coming back to some deep questions about my journey to this place over the last few months.

- Why had it taken so long to come around to the real diagnosis?
- Why had so much time been wasted on the now useless investigation into the "dental" origins of my problem?
- What did God have to do with the late, and now dangerous, diagnosis?
- Did He not want it caught early enough to treat effectively?
- Did He want me to die?

This last question tormented me because I knew this was a serious cancer, and most of the cancer victims that I had known had died.

# CHAPTER 2

# FRIEND OR FOE?

Within a couple of days of the official diagnosis, I was sitting in the examination room of a head and neck cancer specialist. He was a surgeon, and his matter of fact, no-nonsense demeanor caused me to be **more** apprehensive and fearful rather than less. As we discussed my case, I was feeling the same sense of inner despair that I'd had during the conversations with my family doctor. Not that the specialist was himself emotional, or fearful, or anything but pragmatic, for that matter ("realistic" being a big word in cancer care). But, I was deeply affected by the business-like, almost "processed" way he spoke about the disease. He didn't want to speculate until more investigation had been done (made sense to me). He thought an exploratory, day-surgery biopsy procedure (basically "poking around" in my mouth, nasal passages, and throat) was essential in determining the primary tumor site (logical). There wasn't a lot of optimism or pessimism in this part of the discussion, but what tipped the emotional scales for me was the inevitable conversation that all cancer victims have with their first cancer doctor about prognosis.

After the Internet research of the last few days, I had a pretty good idea that the news was going to be bleak. But, I thought that there might be a chance that an ignorant layman like me might have misinterpreted the information, and that a specialist might have something more positive to say (this had generally been my past experience with most doctors). While he continued to be evasive because of early, insufficient knowledge of my personal case, the specialist finally volunteered this statement: **"In my experience, with all comers who have this kind of cancer, about 50% of them are still alive to sit in this room with me after 5 years."** I felt like a few "lifelights" had been snuffed out in my spirit. Fifty percent: That's like someone saying that your life is hanging on one flip of a coin — heads or tails. It was like saying that you are just as likely to lose as to win. Just as likely to die as to live. To anyone but a hopeless gambling addict, fifty percent is dire odds; almost the same as losing, with no second chance to get your money back. The specialist might have sensed some discouragement in my spirit, because he tried to comfort me by adding, "Now remember, fifty percent survival means that about half of my patients are one hundred percent alive after five years (a clever turn of phrase). There's no reason why you aren't going to be one of them." *Was there any reason why I would be one of them?*

There was an unspoken question in this conversation and in many conversations to come. Why, out of a hundred victims with this cancer, would fifty live and fifty die? There are numerous clinical, emotional, and psychological factors that are cited by those who try to explain this statistic. However, for the most part, **it is unknown why the cancer process is different for different people**. It has something to do with the individual, and something to do with the disease. In reality, the bottom line, as I was to learn, is that **they just don't know**. The "fifty percent solution" would become much more significant than I suspected, later on in the journey.

I was scheduled for a CT scan and a surgical biopsy during the following week, and as I walked out of the specialist's office, I felt a strange and powerful sense of my own doom. It was almost like beginning a journey on a path that would take me through numerous, well-meaning people, positive-sounding words, and diligent treatment. But the path would eventually end on an inevitable, no-detour, dead-end street. It was as if both my doctors (so far), while trying to treat me compassionately, were unconsciously preparing me for death whether it be from known or unknown causes. **Even more strange was the incredible pressure on my spirit to see my own death, to accept its inevitability.** I thought, *If the doctors feel powerless to arrest and cure this disease, how are the poor victims supposed to feel?* For the first time in this short, horrific experience, both the deep spiritual fear that I first detected in my family doctor and the cold, hard, "non-spiritual" demeanor of the specialist started to make sense.

For the next several nights, I continued my Internet research on the subject, desperately trying to find a "ray of light" in all the conventional news, clinical trials, and alternative thera-pies. I even looked at a few Christian and secular healing testi-monies. This whole process continued to be discouraging. I was desperately searching for hope while my body, mind, and spirit seemed to be quietly sliding downward.

(*Note: A couple of weeks prior to my diagnosis, I had the opportunity to have lunch with a long-time family friend who had survived colon cancer. He had become very active as a volunteer for the local chapter of the Canadian Cancer Society, and wanted to talk to me about supporting a fund-raising project he was involved with. Interestingly, he also mentioned an alternative, herbal supplement that he was currently taking. He believed that this supplement was a huge factor in his recovery and ongoing protection from cancer. As a further coincidence, a friend of my wife was suspected of having cancer, and so I asked my friend for some information on the herbal supplement. Later, upon learning of my own diagnosis, I immediately thought that God had orchestrated the meeting so that I would learn of the herbal supplement, and that it might hold the key to my own healing. I immediately ordered a 3-month supply of the supplement in the hope that it was a healing gift from God.)*

Although I have related a lot of descriptive physical history, by no means was I spending less time on my spiritual struggle through all of this. From the first suspicion of cancer, I was praying, questioning, and communicating with God in my traditional way, trying to understand what was going on in my life. I had immediately sensed the hand of God in my dilemma, and not necessarily in a good way. I had long believed (in my way) that God was sovereign and in complete control of everything, either by commission (making things happen) or permission (allowing things to happen). And so, for some reason, He was allowing cancer (not, please God, **causing** cancer) to afflict me. Early on, I had prayed for "no cancer," then later for lymphoma (the "good kind" of cancer). Then, upon learning of the actual nature of my disease, I was left with the disturbing notion that not only had God allowed cancer to occur in my life, but an especially serious cancer in the bargain. And this in spite of the many positive and affirming "signals" that He had been sending me throughout the past couple of years. Under other circumstances, this would be merely perplexing. But now, in my situation, it was actually life and death; physically, and perhaps spiritually, too. How much could I have misunderstood Him through all this? What was He up to? Was He teaching me, disciplining me, or judging me?

# CHAPTER 3

# FIRST WORDS

About a week before I was scheduled for my exploratory surgery, a couple of remarkable things happened. I can remember how, at the time, my cynical, struggling mind wondered (or perhaps hoped) that the two events were divinely connected. I had no idea how truly connected they were.

For the past couple of years, Lori had been attending a charismatic Catholic church, and she had become very involved in the spiritual life of this community. This in itself is a fairly lengthy story, so I won't even start to tell it. But, to directly connect Lori's history to my own story, her parish priest had been informed that a U.S.-based healing ministry called "**Whole Life Ministries**" (Augusta Georgia), led by Dr. Sandra Kennedy, was holding meetings in our city over the next few days. Prior to my diagnosis, the priest had given Lori the literature about the ministry, thinking that she might know someone who would benefit, particularly from the ministry's success rate with **cancer healing**. He had passed out the literature, as well, to several parishioners who were dealing with cancer. They included two acquaintances of Lori's: one man who had Hodgkin's lymphoma, and another stricken with a rare form of male breast cancer. Lori and I both considered it more than a coincidence that the priest had passed the information on to us before we knew of my diagnosis. And so, we felt strongly led to attend one of the meetings later that week.

That same night, I began reading my Bible in a kind of random, page-scanning mode. The process was a loose combination of leafing through sections, page by page, as well as occasionally opening to a brand new section, letting my eyes move naturally to areas of the text. I realize that this kind of "laissez faire" approach is frowned upon by many serious Bible readers. In my way, I was hoping for some divine "guidance" or wisdom to help me through this incredible life-and-death situation. I had no spiritual plan, and I realized that searching the Scriptures like this might be an act of desperation born of weak faith. However true this impression might have been, I was still some time removed from the future realization of just how weak my faith in God was.

During this first "open-Bible reading"(as I will refer to it from now on), my eyes came to rest on **Isaiah 30:20-22.**

- **Although the Lord gives you the bread of adversity and the water of affliction, your teachers will be hidden no more; with your own eyes you will see them. Whether you turn to the right or to the left, your ears will hear a voice behind you, saying, "This is the way; walk in it." Then you will defile your idols overlaid with silver and your images covered with gold; you will throw them away like a menstrual cloth and say to them, "Away with you!"**

I can't say exactly how I stumbled upon these verses. Perhaps it was because they were at the top of a page, or more likely, because the opening words of this text were so significant: **"Although the Lord gives you the bread of adversity and the water of affliction..."** I was drawn to this text emotionally (and spiritually, as I realized later on), and was further affected by the next few words: **"your teachers will be hidden no more; with your own eyes you will see them…"** I was immediately struck by the weird, coincidental relationship between this chance Bible discovery and the recent information about Sandra Kennedy's healing meetings. I was still too darkened in my mind to truly embrace the connection, but there was a tiny, mustard-seed of faith that hoped it was a kind of confirmation of the relationship. I shared the text with Lori and tucked it away in the "questions to be answered later" compartment of my heart.

The second connective event originated from another direction. We had planned to attend the second day of the Kennedy meetings, and on the evening before that day, we received a phone call from a relative of Lori, who was aware of my situation. By way of quick background, he had recently experienced what looked dangerously like a major epileptic seizure. He had just undergone the requisite CT scan and EEG protocol to determine the cause and was awaiting the results. Although a sincere Christian believer, he was not a particularly active churchgoer, but he had called to tell us about something interesting he had experienced the day before. On a bit of a whim, he had attended Sandra Kennedy's healing meeting on the previous night, and during the service he had received a deep, sudden conviction from God that he was healed. Being that he was a lawyer by profession and very pragmatic, almost cynical by nature, this "word" from God was all the more remarkable to him. So remarkable, in fact, that he called us to suggest that we might want to attend one of Dr. Kennedy's meetings. *(Note: A few days later, his tests all came back normal. However, a few months later on, he experienced a recurrent seizure episode, and was re-diagnosed with a milder form of epilepsy. Although he now takes medication to prevent future occurrences, we continue to stand in faith on the original "healing word" he received that day.)* You can imagine how this phone call intrigued me, when combined with the Isaiah text and the initial receipt of the meeting information from the priest. These events had subtly implanted a small seed of hope in my darkened, frightened, wholly human heart. The following day, we attended the meeting with a heightened sense of interest and mystery.

I arrived at the meeting on my own, expecting Lori to arrive separately from her place of work. I was quite early, so the sanctuary of the hosting church was still fairly empty, with people steadily filing in. I found a pew about halfway up the aisle, sat down and reflected on my situation. Since my conversion to Christianity, I had believed in God's discretionary power to heal, and in fact, believed that He had been the key to my healing from chronic fatigue syndrome some 15 years earlier. In spite of this personal "healing" experience, the passage of time, as well as the fact that we were now dealing with CANCER, had left me with more questions than answers, more doubts than assurance. Furthermore, I hadn't known anyone who had been healed of cancer. God could make the lame walk, the blind see, and the chronically fatigued well, but He didn't seem to be very effective with cancer; maybe fifty percent of the time, if the statistics were to be believed. As I mentioned before, this percentage was to become very important later on. Still, I was hoping to be hit by a holy, healing "bolt of lightning" at this meeting, or at least get a "word" like our relative had received the night before.

As I waited for Lori, more people started to file in. While there were still plenty of empty pews, a couple stopped next to my row and asked if they could sit in the pew that I was occupying. I politely let them in, and we sat together in reflective silence, until I spotted Lori entering the room. As she approached the pew, I noticed her waving a greeting in my general direction, but not directly at me. I then saw the woman next to me waving "hello" at Lori, and I felt puzzled to be sure. They obviously knew each other. It turned out that this couple attended the same catholic church that Lori went to, and the husband was the one I mentioned earlier who had been recently diagnosed with a rare form of male breast cancer. He had just undergone surgery to remove the tumor and was now scheduled for chemotherapy. While we were still reeling from this weird rendezvous, the other gentleman from Lori's church, the one with Hodgkin's lymphoma, showed up and joined us in the pew. There we were, all five of us; just a coincidence upon a coincidence.

Sandra Kennedy's ministry is just one of many healing ministries active in North American Christianity. We all know that divine healing is one of the most controversial subjects today for believers and non-believers alike. It is not helpful that, through the years, some healing ministries have been discredited as being nothing more than fraudulent, religious entertainment. So, for many Christians, divine healing remains a mystery that most hope they will never have to seek. But for those of us sitting there waiting for the meeting to start, we felt that we had somehow been brought there for a reason.

Dr. Kennedy's approach is somewhat different than the conventional prayer line, "laying on of hands" healing ministry (although she does lay hands on the sick at the end of her meetings). Her main healing gift (I believe) is expressed first, through the diligent preaching of the biblical message, affirming God's general will to heal all of us. Then, she teaches and exhorts us to believe that God's healing can be received as a personal word of healing for the individual. And finally, she encourages seekers to pray for the Holy Spirit's guidance and enabling to receive this personal *rhema* word from God. *(Note: "rhema" is one of the original Greek terms used to define a variant of the term "word" as it appears in the Bible. It is used to describe very specific, personal messages from God that are "spoken" or "uttered" to an individual. These "rhema" words carry an individual, targeted message for that person alone. This meaning differs from the use of the Greek term "logos," which denotes the "word" as a medium for the universal knowledge of the will or intent of God, applicable to believers in general.)* Dr. Kennedy teaches that God's personal will for us can be discerned and then connected with through hearing or reading Scriptures which uniquely speak to our situation **("... faith comes by hearing, and hearing by the Word of God" — Romans 10:17).** As opposed to believing that all Scripture can be "made to fit" our situation, or believing that merely reciting or memorizing healing Scripture texts will be effective, **Dr. Kennedy believes that God will speak directly to us through the Word, with a healing promise meant specifically for us.** She is convinced that the Holy Spirit will prompt us with a deep-seated conviction in our hearts when we are given such a *rhema* word. When this conviction occurs, "we will know that we know that we know that God has healed us" (her words).

During the meeting, her message was organized, engaging, and biblically sound. There was none of the euphoria or "theatrics" one might associate with certain well-known healing evangelists. *(Note: One very important feature of her teaching is affirming the practical cooperation between modern medical treatment and God's supernatural power to heal.)* However, all throughout the teaching and prayer time, some people were declaring their healing by a show of raised hands or by exclaiming, "I got it!" I was waiting, and quietly hoping for something to happen, even though I knew that I was still skeptical. By the end of the meeting, I couldn't say "that I knew that I knew that I knew" anything, but her teaching had struck a tiny chord of truth inside my doubting heart. This chord continued to resonate over the next few days, even as I prepared myself for surgery and treatment.

That same weekend, I sent e-mail letters to my two closest, faith communities: my church and the Convergence radio team. *(Note: For over two years I had been the executive producer of an offbeat, Christian radio program called "Convergence Café." The program had a "reality" format, with original drama, music, and spoken word. We were blessed to be on the air in Western Canada for the two years previous to my cancer diagnosis.)* I had already spoken personally to my immediate family, my four sisters, my four most intimate friends, and my two pastors. But the sheer number of people who would notice my abrupt absence from church and radio duties was just too large (80-plus) for me to effectively engage, so I e-mailed them. In addition, while I had told my personal family members and confidantes the full extent of my cancer diagnosis, I had decided not to detail this in the general e-letters. Instead, I informed everyone of my regretful, forced absence, which would extend for an indeterminate period of time, while I was dealing with a "serious illness." I made no mention of the word "cancer." I expressed my love for everyone and asked for prayer. I chose this path of keeping a very close, private circle of confidence for a couple of reasons. As time unfolded, I became increasingly convinced that this was the most correct and spiritually wise course for my own journey. Here's why.

- From the beginning of the "trial by fire," I had a deep conviction that I would need to devote all my heart, mind, and spirit to understand it and hopefully to overcome it, as God had evidently allowed it to happen. By keeping the number of informed people to a minimum, I hoped to avoid having to engage too many people, at too many levels, when news of my "condition" spread. It was the most important issue of my entire life, and I didn't feel everyone had a right to know. I had always been an intensely private person, and I hoped God would understand and show me somehow that this was OK.

- One significant point in Sandra Kennedy's teaching on healing was **the influence of the faith of others on the afflicted person's healing outcome.** This effect was explained from an intercessory prayer perspective and from an authentic encouragement perspective. Dr. Kennedy's very sound advice was to be extremely careful and selective in choosing people to confide in, to pray with you, or to walk beside you in such an important spiritual ordeal. Her contention was that, although many Christians *say* they believe that God heals today, many of those same Christians do not *really* believe it. In addition, there are many who will tell you outright that they don't believe it, or that perhaps they believe God will heal only in some randomized, mysterious way. This mindset seems to be especially true of cancer, where, for many believers, prayer seems like a pitifully weak weapon against such a formidable disease. In fact, the unspoken presumption of death and defeat can sometimes transform "well meaning" comments, attitudes, and prayers into a negative spiritual force. This negative force can be a factor where faith in God's Word is not an authentic foundation, but merely a façade. I was having enough problems struggling with my own faith in the matter, and I didn't want to contend with anyone else's struggle, however well meaning. So, I reasoned that people might pray more positively if they did not know it was cancer. I hoped that God would bring forth a few trusted, believing individuals who could pray and believe in faith for my healing, **knowing** that it was cancer. I hoped that I would be one of them.

That same weekend I spent some more time doing open Bible reading, and again I found myself in the book of Isaiah where my eyes came to rest on **Isaiah 41:8-24.**

- The opening words, **"But you, O Israel, my servant, Jacob, whom I have chosen...."** (Isaiah 41:8), seemed to speak to that place in my heart that had always longed to be "chosen," to be special.
- As I read further in this passage, I was somewhat encouraged as I read words like, **"I have chosen you and have not rejected you....do not fear, for I am with you....I will strengthen you....I will uphold you with My righteous right hand"**(Isaiah 41: 9, 10). I was feeling that kind of generic encouragement that most Christians feel when they read such words that are universal and timeless but not particularly personal.
- As I read on, the encouragement increased a little as the text spoke, **"All who rage against you will surely be ashamed and disgraced; those who oppose you will be as nothing and perish"** (Isaiah 41:11). I wistfully imagined "all those who rage" to be the cancer that had invaded my body.
- Then, the next words intrigued me even more: **"Though you search for your enemies, you will not find them... Those who wage war against you will be as nothing at all"** (Isaiah 41:12). Were the doctors not searching for my enemy, the primary tumor? I had been told that, for cases of "squamous cell carcinoma of occult (unknown) origin," about fifty percent of the time the primary tumor is not found, and that this often improves survival time. This was due to the tumor being too small (and perhaps too slow growing) to be immediately dangerous. Perhaps this scripture was meaningful after all. Could it mean that the doctors would not find the primary tumor and thus, my chances of living longer would be improved due to it being a smaller tumor? Could it mean that God would somehow render the cancerous lymph nodes suddenly misdiagnosed or harmless?

The next words continued to be encouraging, especially **"See, I will make you into a threshing sledge, new and sharp, with many teeth" (Isaiah 41:15).** The "I will" part seemed to talk about a future of restoration and new purpose.

As I read on, the words of restoration and blessing continued down the page. And just when I had determined that my positive thinking session had kind of "petered out," my heart was stunned by the next passage. **"Present your case," says the Lord." Set forth your arguments," says Jacob's King. "Bring in your idols to tell us what is going to happen. Tell us what the former things were, so that we may consider them and know their final outcome. Or declare to us the things to come, tell us what the future holds, so we may know that you are gods. Do something, whether good or bad, so that we will be dismayed and filled with fear. But you are less than nothing, and your works are utterly worthless; he who chooses you is detestable" (Isaiah 41:21-24).**

As I read this text, I was overwhelmed with images of my recent consultations with doctors; my intensive Internet research into cancer facts and statistics; and, my attitudes and responses to them all. I couldn't help thinking that this ancient Bible text was describing, in some detail, what I had been experiencing.

- **"Tell us what the former things were, so that we may know their final outcome..."** i.e., the results of previous cancer studies; cancer statistics. They were dependable, clinical data for predicting the future.
- **"...tell us what the future holds, so that we may know you are gods."** We often hang on every word from our doctor as if it comes from "on high."
- **"Do something, whether good or bad, so that we will be dismayed and filled with fear."** With cancer, any consultation or clinical result is subject to qualifications, even-

tual error, or failure. Even "good news" is conditional, and consequently, fear never really leaves the scene.

I couldn't shake the feeling that I was actually "inside" this ancient Bible passage; **that it was actually describing my situation.** Perhaps God somehow wanted it to speak to me. Could this be what Sandra Kennedy meant by a *rhema* word? The question now began to "hang there," permanently on the mindscape.

The story began to unfold more dramatically over the next few days. In response to my e-mails, I began to receive numerous messages of love, support, and prayer from my faith communities. One message in particular revolved around the encouraging exhortation, **"Gather your strength, mighty warrior,"** complete with a scanned picture of a warrior battling a dragon. A couple of days later, my open Bible reading took me to **Judges 6 and 7, the story of Gideon.** As I read the opening few verses of the story, where it describes the oppression of Israel by the Midianites, my heart stirred again over the word pictures that had been chosen by the writer of the text.

- **The Lord ... gave them into the hands of the Midianites. Because the power of Midian was so oppressive...Whenever the Israelites planted their crops, the Midianites... invaded the country. They camped on the land and ruined the crops...and did not spare a living thing...They came up with their livestock and their tents like swarms of locusts. It was impossible to count the men and their camels; they invaded the land to ravage it. Midian so impoverished the Israelites that they cried out to the Lord for help (Judges 6:1-6).** I was overwhelmed, again, by the mental image of cancer doing the same thing to my body and to the bodies of other victims. The disease was invading, multiplying, spreading, overwhelming, oppressing, terrorizing, and killing. I couldn't help asking myself if God was giving me a Biblical picture of the disease that was attacking me.

- As I read on in the text, I learned that the invasion had something to do with the Israelites' disobedience in turning to other gods. **I said to you, "I am the Lord your God; do not worship the gods of the Amorites *[Baal and Asherah]*, in whose land you live." But you have not listened to me" (Judges 6:10).**

- Then I experienced the first of many stunned reactions when I read: **Gideon was <u>threshing wheat</u>...When the angel of the Lord appeared to Gideon, he said, "The Lord is with you, <u>mighty warrior</u>" (Judges 6:11-12).**

  - **"threshing wheat"** — Didn't the Isaiah 41 scripture I had read previously say that the Lord would make Jacob (Israel) into "a threshing sledge, new and sharp"?
  - **"mighty warrior"** — Hadn't my friend just sent me a message calling me by the same title? Why was my heart stirring so much? Did these coincidental connections between my "random" scripture readings and the recent correspondence from other people mean anything, spiritually or otherwise?

Even in my stressed, fearful state, I couldn't deny the feeling that I was on the threshold of some kind of mystery. I read the rest of the story of Gideon and his divine calling to deliver Israel from the Midianites. It is truly an incredible story, full of faith and victory. But, I wouldn't allow myself to believe that this story could also be about me and my own war with cancer. I mean, who wants (or dares) to compare himself, other than symbolically or humorously, with any great man of God? Especially considering that someone like myself had so much to regret and confess. But, the "threshing" connection and the title "mighty warrior" compelled me to keep this discovery tucked away in my heart for future reference. My skeptical nature caused me to presume that my friend had actually been pointing me to the story of Gideon by using the term "mighty warrior." I was sure that he assumed I would know where the reference came from. Although I had casually read the story a couple of times in the past, I definitely did not recall that title being used.

If my friend had actually been prompted by the story of Gideon, it would diminish the likelihood that this connection was due to any kind of special guidance "from God's hand." In other words, who would believe that I had just "accidentally fallen" into the book of Judges and "stumbled over" the same title used in my friend's e-mail? I **had** to know, so I immediately e-mailed him and asked him where he had obtained the inspiration to call me a "mighty warrior." Surprisingly, he replied with a lengthy message, explaining his image of my medical battle, with me as a warrior, joined by other prayer warriors, engaged in a dramatic, physical and spiritual conflict. He had decidedly **not** used Gideon as an inspiration, and so now I was beginning to believe in the possibility that God had orchestrated this weird connection. Even though the story of Gideon continues on to describe some amazing exploits of idol-busting and military victory, I didn't want to get too ahead of myself (or God) by over-thinking this new "coincidence." Besides, at this moment, I wasn't capable of much more than just coping with my situation and concentrating on "gettin' healed," as Sandra Kennedy would say. The hopeful part in "receiving" all of this new Scripture information was that there was a **future** spoken of. I hung on to this hope of a future with all my strength.

# CHAPTER 4

# VOICES

I want to talk a little about hearing God through "voices." By this I don't mean the audible, "burning bush"-type voices, but instead "hearing" voices with your mind and heart. I know that the concept of "hearing God" is well accepted in most Christian circles. For those who have that kind of special relationship with the Lord, we are often told of God actually communicating with them (for instance, " God spoke to me about…" or, "God told me to…"). I am not a person to whom God has "spoken" much. The problem is usually mine, as I often wonder (maybe you do too) if what I "hear" in my head is just my own rendering of what I think God might say, or worse, what I want God to say. Yet, I can confirm a few, very significant moments in my life where I am convinced God did speak to me. I believe this mainly because the words, or statements, were communicated in such a way that it didn't really sound like something I would think, let alone say; it was as if they had a structure and style difference. So, I reasoned that if it didn't "sound" like me, then it was more likely to be God.

One major handicap you encounter when you learn you have cancer is that your mind and emotions go into a kind of zone which feels like everything is in overdrive. Sleeping is difficult, your sensitivities to almost everything change, and your mind works overtime. You think constantly about your situation, treatment, prognosis, death, options, hopes, and God. New and unexpected thoughts just pop into your mind. So, in some ways, you feel even more on your guard about actually hearing from God, especially because you so much **want** to hear from Him. **Smith Wigglesworth**, the great, early 20th century evangelist wrote: **"I want to warn you of the foolishness of listening to voices…Look in the Bible…Don't run away with anything else…If you hear a (legitimate) voice it will be in line with the scriptures of truth from the Word of God"** (*Ever Increasing Faith*, **Gospel Publishing House, c. 1924**). This very logical advice from Wigglesworth would prove to be a dependable anchor throughout the journey, because, frankly, I contended with "voices" (audible thoughts, I guess) on a fairly continuous basis. And, I continually tried to test these voices against the general principles of Scripture as well as the elements of *rhema* scripture that I would be progressively led to. Without going into a complete transcript of the "voice" portion of my journey, I will give you a couple of examples of what I heard and the resulting faith dilemma this led to. Again, this can happen because we want so much to hear something, anything.

First, it may be helpful to illustrate the two basic categories of "voice" that I contended with.

-   You will recall that, early on in my diagnosis, I had purchased a three-month supply of my family friend's recommended, alternative cancer cure, which was an herbal supplement (name withheld). I had been taking it for a few days, hoping that the coincidental nature of its discovery represented something truly meaningful. Then one afternoon, quite abruptly, as I was about to swallow a capsule, I heard what amounted to a kind of shout in

my head: **"Stop taking (name withheld)!"** It was so
loud that I almost dropped the capsule, and, at the same
time, I felt a distinct conviction to obey the voice. At the
time, it seemed quite irrational. A couple of future, spiritual discoveries would later validate this voice, but for
that moment, it took a lot of my will to cooperate. This
was particularly because I had not yet read the Smith
Wigglesworth statement, and especially because I was so
fearful of my disease. Yet, I still stopped the supplement,
because something in my spirit just seemed to affirm it.

- The second example is a little more complicated,
because it begins with what I came to recognize as the
"voice of the enemy." I think that all human beings think
about the general concept of death from time to time,
and throughout life, it's probably quite normal to think
**occasionally** about one's own death. Upon learning of
my cancer diagnosis, I often found myself preoccupied with thoughts, visions, daydreams, and musings
about the circumstances surrounding my "impending"
death. Sometimes I would experience the abject fear of
picturing myself wasting away and suffering horribly.
Sometimes I would catch myself imagining scenes
inside the hospital, or even around my bed as I lay dying.
Sometimes I would fall into thinking about details of my
funeral (songs that would be sung, people who might
attend, etc.), or about the distribution of my estate and
finances. Almost every conceivable angle of approach
to my death doggedly hung around me, day and night.
These images and thoughts covered the full spectrum of
emotions, from fearful to almost whimsical. Some of this
preoccupation I attributed to my own darker nature (I
had always thought about death), but the sheer volume
and pervasiveness of these thoughts and daydreams
made me wonder if something else was also at work.
When I wasn't thinking about treatment and healing, I

was thinking about death, and death was winning the battle for my mind. Then one day, as I was in the shower, praying and reflecting, these images of my death began to cascade with increasing momentum inside my mind, and then began to penetrate more deeply into my heart. I began to feel as if I was drowning, about to be overcome. I was so overcome that I quietly but audibly cried out to God. I thought that perhaps this avalanche of thoughts was from Him, trying to tell me to surrender to His will: my death. Standing in the shower I said, **"God, if this is coming from You, do you want me to just give in to these overwhelming thoughts of death?"** Just as immediately, and just as loudly as the first warning about the herbal supplement, I sensed the word **"No!"** literally "shouted" inside my heart. I could almost hear the shout. It was spoken with incredible urgency and power, as if whoever shouted it knew that I was just about to step off a precipice and fall into the abyss. I remember feeling like someone had just slapped me in the face to awaken me from a nightmare. I prayed silently, acknowledging that I would not accept the visions of death, no matter how persuasive they were. And, I would continue to reach for healing and life from God.

At the same time, I began to see a spiritual pattern in this relentless, death-attack on my mind. Theories about the "power of positive thinking" notwithstanding, I was struck by the incredible **"death momentum"** that a cancer diagnosis prompts in its victims. My case may be somewhat extreme, but I could see how the preoccupation with death could begin quite subtly, and, through the course of time, increase its force to the point where one becomes not only quite convinced, but actually resigned to an expected fate. This resignation to the outcome often occurs long before it may actually happen. Another question began to take root. **Could this death**

**momentum begin in the mind, then penetrate the heart, and then, finally overwhelm the spirit, literally making its own reality?** The "shower experience", although very early in the journey, marked a bit of a turning point in my spiritual understanding of cancer. From that moment, I began to assign responsibility for these "daydreams of death" to the enemy, who came **"to steal and kill and destroy" (John 10:10)**. Conversely, I assigned authorship of the shouted "NO!" to the Lord, who wanted me healed and alive.

# CHAPTER 5

# THE FIRST CUT IS (NOT) THE DEEPEST

The day for my exploratory surgery arrived, and in a way, the deep reality of my illness arrived as well. Lori and I drove to the hospital, where we were briefed by the surgeon on the procedure. He was going to "poke around" and take some tissue samples. In addition, we authorized him to perform whatever additional surgery he deemed necessary — whatever that meant. I was wheeled into the operating room, where I suddenly felt overwhelmed by the images of lights, surgical instruments, masked doctors and nurses. As the anesthetic took effect, my feelings were dream-like and resigned. I slipped into an uneasy peace. When I awoke in the recovery room, the surgeon came in and told us that he had removed both my tonsils, and that my right tonsil "looked quite suspicious." During my Internet research, I remembered seeing information on surgery for head and neck cancer (not very pleasant or hopeful material). And so, I asked if the surgical removal of my tonsil would also accomplish the removal of the tumor, if the pathology came back confirming cancer. The surgeon very quickly said "No," that he had just done a very superficial tonsillectomy, and that we would have to wait and see. I was sent home with some painkillers, and with the clear, stark understanding that we had just officially crossed the border from diagnosis into the realm of treatment. The road sign read "Now Entering Cancerville."

For the next two weeks, I recovered from my surgery at home, sleeping in an upright position because my salivary/mucus equilibrium had been upset by the operation. As this weird fluid mixture gathered in my mouth and throat, I would literally choke if I slept lying down. I would become very used to this position over the next few months. I popped the painkillers, rested, reflected, prayed, and made ready to learn more about my specific condition and treatment. Right from the beginning I had spent a lot of time focusing, with all of my senses, on dealing with my new life inside cancer. The fact that I was in some pain, and needed to rest, merely added to the opportunity to sit, think, and pray about my situation. About a week after surgery, I learned that the surgeon's suspicion was correct; a confirmed, primary tumor in my right tonsil.

I immediately went to the Internet again, zeroing in on information for my type and stage of cancer. Once again, the prognosis suggested was not any more optimistic than before: about 50/50. I was so discouraged by this clinical information that I once again began to surf for sites with cancer healing stories, miracles, and other Christian perspectives on cancer. Although these websites were not very definitive medically and statistically, they provided the only sense of real hope to my brutalized, vulnerable, and very small faith. I thought that I had always believed in divine healing. In fact, I had publicly attributed my healing from chronic fatigue to God, with the secondary help of Chinese herbs, exercise, and mega-vitamins. I thought that I believed, until I realized that I mostly believed in a detached, "observer" kind of way. Sure, God healed people … people with legendary, unshakeable faith (not me) ... people who could pray with righteousness and integrity (not me) ... people who deserved healing (not me). I realized that even though I talked about divine healing, I had placed a lot more faith in herbs, homeopathy, vitamins, and daily exercise to keep me healthy. I had more faith in the remedies than I did in the God of the universe. I was not really a spiritual fake, but more of a spiritual weakling. I believed in God, in His provision for salvation, in His power to chasten or punish me, and even in His power to heal me, but not in His **desire** to heal me. Perhaps my doubt was because I had been stricken with "The Big One:" cancer; and especially, because **God had allowed it to be *my* cancer.** In spite of these disabling doubts, my last bit of Internet research convinced me to do two things that would change the course of the journey, and ultimately change my life (praise God). **First, I decided to completely stop all Internet research on the clinical, factual, and statistical world of cancer. It was all about death anyway. And second, I decided to try and understand (and maybe believe) the biblical mystery of God's healing provision.**

I was clearly no biblical scholar, nor even a regular Bible reader. There were, however, a couple of anecdotes involving Bible words in the original Greek that encouraged me to seek knowledge about God's healing will.

- The first anecdote was an explanation of the word "save" as spoken in the New Testament by Jesus and the apostles. I had heard this explanation for the first time within Sandra Kennedy's messages. The word "save" is translated from the Greek word *sozo*, which carries with it a much broader meaning than most lay Christians are normally led to believe. In addition to the spiritual salvation meaning of *sozo*, the Greek word also describes saving a person through the **healing of the body and mind as well**. A more complete salvation, if you will.

- The second anecdote involves my own Bible reading journey, where on a certain evening I remembered the passage in **2Timothy 1:7 (NKJ): "For God has not given us a spirit of fear, but of power and of love and of a sound mind."** I also remembered that the word "power" had a meaningful, Greek root word as well. After a little research, I found that the Greek word for power was *dunamis* (we get our words dynamite and dynamic from this root). Since the Bible stated that we had been given this spirit of *dunamis*, I used a concordance (very scholarly of me) to find some other references to "power" in the Bible. One passage that stood out was **Isaiah 11:2, a well known, Old Testament prophecy about Jesus Christ: "The Spirit of the Lord will rest on him == the Spirit of wisdom and of understanding, the Spirit of counsel and of power, the Spirit of knowledge and of the fear of the Lord."** I was a little startled to find out that the Greek word for "power" in this Old Testament reference to Jesus was, in fact, *dunamis* as well, which meant that we had been given **the same Spirit of power as Jesus** had been given.

These little bytes of knowledge didn't transform my faith exactly, but they did increase my resolve to discover if the "truth" that I had always "parroted" to friends and family was, in fact, **THE TRUTH**. It's amazing how the fascinating, theo-philosophical questions of life and death so urgently require concrete answers when facing the **reality** of life and death.

# CHAPTER 6

# ITEM #1: JESUS

My first step toward discovering this Truth was to read and evaluate all the New Testament accounts of Jesus' healing ministry. *(Note: An important reminder to the reader is that my evaluation of Scripture passages was by no means a formal, scholarly analysis [original languages, historical context, or supplementary commentaries]. Normally, I did not utilize any resources other than what was already contained in the footnotes of my study Bible. I say this because, whatever impressions or meaning that I perceived from my Bible reading occurred in a natural, often spontaneous, and decidedly non-intellectual manner. I engaged the Scriptures without a lot of predisposition or prejudice, other than a very shallow belief in their potential truth.)* I was able to find approximately forty accounts of Jesus' healing activity in the four Gospels. As I read each account, I allowed my mental painting of His healing ministry to gather form, color, and detail. Very quickly I was confronted with a key decision that we all have to make when we speak of the dynamics of divine healing: **I had to decide if it is really God's will to heal us.** This question of "God's will" is the pendulum that swings between two images of God.

- The first is the image of a God who wants us to know and understand Him most of the time (predictability or dependability).
- The second is the image of a God who is unknowable except for the sheer awe we experience at His mystery (unpredictability). Sandra Kennedy had an interesting way of expressing this issue when she said (and I paraphrase), **"If one does not believe in God's general will to heal everyone, then we make God into a scary God, or even a bad God, because "you never know what God's gonna do."**

I realized that for years I had been "faithfully" praying healing prayers for people in this very conditional way; "Lord, please heal (name), **if it be Your will.**" It sounds so spiritual and obedient when you say it this way. Even Jesus seemed to pray this kind of prayer in Gethsemane when He asked, in **Luke 22:42, "Father, if you are willing, take this cup from me; yet not my will, but yours be done."** (Of course, He already **KNEW** what the Father's will was). In our world, this prayer qualifier of **"if it be Your will"** also suggests a kind of "safety zone" for uncertain faith when it's applied to typical petitionary prayers. If we qualify our petitions with this safe phrase, then the various, alternate outcomes of such prayers need not be seen as any significant comment on our personal faith. In other words, regardless of what we specifically prayed for, we fully accommodated any outcome, because any outcome was probably God's will.

I knew about the perennial debate over God's healing will, and I counted myself among the millions of Christians who cannot, by experience, validate divine healing very much, if at all. One practical question that haunted me very early in the journey was whether or not it was God's perfect will that so many cancer victims (50% overall) eventually died of the disease. My examination of the scriptural accounts of Jesus' healing ministry only added to, rather than detracted from, this controversy.

As I read and re-read the forty-or-so Gospel accounts of Jesus' healing of the sick, I became amazed at the richness and the depth of His healing character. Each text contributed to making my image of Jesus more real, more complete, more believable. His healing provision, in each situation, was demonstrated in a way that seemed to evaluate and adapt to all of our very human inconsistencies.

- **Jesus healed <u>every</u> disease and sickness (Matthew 4:23).**
- **When asked if He was willing, <u>He was</u> (Matthew 8:1-3).**
- **Jesus was <u>willing to go out of His way</u> to heal, but would also <u>heal from a distance </u>with just a word (Matthew 8:5-13).**
- **He healed when He saw someone had <u>faith</u> (Matthew 9:1-8).**
- **He healed spontaneously when someone <u>touched Him</u> (Matthew 9:18-26).**
- **He stopped to heal when He heard <u>the sick cry out to Him</u> (Matthew 9:27-30).**
- **He had <u>compassion</u> for the sick and helpless <u>which moved Him to heal</u> (Matthew 9:35-36).**
- **He responded to <u>persistence</u>, even flippancy from the needy (Matthew 15:21-28).**
- **He healed <u>all who came</u> to Him (Matthew 21:14-15).**
- **He healed <u>those brought</u> to Him (Mark 1:29-34).**

This evidence of the multi-dimensional nature of Jesus' healing ministry pointed toward **His demonstrated, general will to heal all who were in His "circle of awareness."** My heart was stirring at this thought. So, how high, wide, deep, or infinite is that circle of awareness? That was a rhetorical question if I ever heard one. In point of fact, the only account which described a limitation or condition upon Jesus' "demonstrated will" to heal was in **Mark 6:1-6,** where He entered a town and later departed, having only healed a few people, because **He was so "amazed at their lack of faith."** This scripture raised some new questions to ponder:

- How serious is an unbelief or doubt that causes Jesus to be amazed?
- What kind of human condition would be significant enough, or stunning enough to "amaze" the God of the Universe?
- Is God "amazed" by normal, human doubt?
- Does this Scripture imply that our common, human struggle with disbelief or doubt is enough to block God's healing will?

If the answer to the last question is "Yes," then this is a very simple explanation for our countless failures to receive divine healing. Oh, did I mention that it also is a very effective tool of discouragement and abuse for many believers. ("He didn't receive healing because he lacked faith; unbelief killed him.") I know that this sounds harsh, but it's the "blemish that won't go away" in our struggle to understand the truth of divine healing. Do all those afflicted people who prayed for healing, but didn't receive it, suffer from the kind of unbelief that literally "amazes" God into inactivity or even disability? Or is there a deeper explanation? Trying to pinpoint your theoretical position on the "faith and belief grid" is an interesting, even stimulating, exercise when you're healthy. It's much different when you realize that your actual position may determine life or death.

Once I came to an intellectual knowledge of Jesus' demonstrated will to heal, there was another key question that clearly needed an answer. It had to do with how this knowledge really meant anything to me today, now, in my own situation. Again, I remembered some scriptures that addressed this question, at least, from a theological standpoint, that is.

- **"And surely I am with you always, to the very end of the age" (Matthew 28:20).**
- **"Jesus Christ is the same yesterday and today and forever" (Hebrews 13:8).**
- **"If you really knew Me, you would know My Father as well" (John 14:7).**
- **"Anyone who has seen Me has seen the Father" (John 14:9).**

We've already seen how Jesus, while on Earth, had a demonstrated healing will. Now, according to these scriptures above (and numerous others), whether incarnated or forever resurrected as Christ, or in His unity with the Father, **Jesus was demonstrating a healing will that was, by scriptural definition, also <u>God's healing will.</u> Following** these steps of logic, through Bible study, encouraged me and raised my hopes, but my inherent skepticism kept me from immediately adopting this connection as the Truth. After all, lots of sick people (and their intercessors) claimed to believe this important truth, and yet many still suffered and died, which raised the whole question again about God's will. (This cycle can make your head hurt.) **On the other hand, if it *was* the Truth, then what was blocking or preventing people from connecting with God's (demonstrated) desire to heal them?** Even if I could not completely believe in the concept I had just studied in the Scriptures, it certainly whetted my appetite to try and understand more. I had a sincere desire to find some clue to connect me with God's healing will.There had to be a reason why so many people with cancer seemed excluded from, or were unable to receive, the healing that

God apparently wanted to give. There had to be a reason. Cancer seemed to be such a formidable — even invincible — disease.

As I recovered from my tonsil surgery, I spent a lot of time struggling with thoughts of suffering, death, eternity, my past, God's will for me, and the mysterious truth of the Bible. I had always called the Bible "The Word of God," but I knew that I was being challenged to stand my ground or else retreat from that definition. I seemed to have an easier time believing the Bible's promises about eternity than I did believing the concept of God's power to heal in "the here and now." (Even though I believed that I had experienced a form of this healing some fifteen years previous.) I now see that my real issue was "half-believing," or somehow being afraid to completely believe.This struggle had the effect of reminding me that it was impossible to believe in only "selected" aspects of the Bible. If we could pick and choose what we wanted to believe (as many "believers" do), then we would leave ourselves open to never really knowing what is the absolute Truth. This selective uncertainty could threaten even that which we think we solidly believe in, like salvation for instance. Even my belief in salvation was weaker than I thought, as I struggled with my fear of death on a relatively continual basis. However, I am also convinced that even this weak "salvation faith" at least kept me in the battle to receive additional faith to engage God's Word.

I fought this "mind battle" for days and nights. Every time I sensed myself moving toward greater faith in what I had learned so far, my thoughts would always be punctuated with the whispering reminder, *But remember, it's cancer.* I alternated between believing that this was Satan whispering to me and believing that it was just my own darkened memories of the power of cancer in the natural world. Either way, the whispers were currently my worst enemy.

# CHAPTER 7

# THE REAL ENEMY MEETS HOPE

A few days before my first official treatment consultation at the cancer clinic, I had a telephone conversation. It was an awakening, really, that changed everything.
One of the priorities of this very private ordeal was to seek
God's guidance in gathering a small group of confidantes. It
was to be a group with whom details of my illness could be
shared, and most importantly, with whom Lori and I could
pray with, and be prayed for, in faith. As I mentioned much
earlier in this account, the determination of who would be
in this group was not as easy as you might think, especially
because it involved "THE BIG C." Although I knew that
there were many people of my acquaintance who possessed
faith larger than mine, I wondered: Did that larger faith apply
to cancer?

About twenty years earlier, we had met a couple at the
hospital at the time of the births of our first children. We had
maintained contact with them for a few years, lost contact for
another few, and then, quite miraculously, had reconnected
with them again about thirteen years ago. They are a truly
remarkable couple. Don is functionally deaf, a self-employed
professional engineer, and although unable to hear well,

he possesses incredibly attuned spiritual hearing. His wife, Hope, was born with cerebral palsy, and had been divinely healed of this condition some thirteen years earlier during a worship service at their church. Hope had been a very close prayer partner and friend to Lori throughout the last few years of our marriage. I also learned that she had recently experienced a vision of my late mother. In the vision, my mother had asked Hope to "be there for my son and daughter-in-law." After some emotional discussions with Lori about appropriate prayer partners for my situation, I decided to call Hope personally. I wanted to see what God might do in our conversation to provide some sign that she and Don were being raised up to pray with us. Given their life histories, I anticipated that there was not too much lacking on the "faith front" for healing, especially in Hope's case, but I was in for an incredible shock. As it turns out, a holy shock.

I wasn't prepared for the response I would get when I asked Hope about her faith and her willingness to pray with us for healing and restoration from cancer. I want to say that this conversation was not some kind of qualification test or "third degree." I was painfully aware of my own weak faith for this coming ordeal, constantly under attack with doubts and death thoughts. I think what I was looking for was an assurance that healing faith was possible in other people, and hence, possible for me. As we talked on the phone, Hope surprised me when we reached the central reason for the call. Rather than just speaking words of faith and support, she began to tell me a story of her personal scarring at the hands of the cancer monster.

Her father had died of cancer in spite Hope's fervent, faith-filled prayers, as well as those of many other loving intercessors. For years Hope had harbored a secret fear, a defeatist fear, of praying for people with cancer. This was not only because of her father, but because of the accumulated experience of seeing so many fellow believers suffer and die from the disease (sound familiar?). This dread of the power of cancer had actually caused her to first secretly, then openly, *avoid praying* for the healing of cancer victims. This was sadly ironic, for she was often called upon to pray for sick people as a "divinely healed person" herself. When asked to pray for cancer victims, she opted (safely) instead to pray for comfort, grace, or peace for the victim and the family. These were faith prayers to be sure, but they masked the deep hurt she felt in the presence of a God who seemed to heal everything *but* cancer. Hope even alluded to the secret fear that many of us harbor as well, which is that, even in the face of faithful prayer and petition, cancer is the one disease that God appears to have a mysterious "indifference" toward, or at least some unknown "reluctance" to heal. In this very emotional conversation, Hope then went on to describe a series of encounters with God that had prepared her, as she quoted Scripture, **"for such a time as this" (Esther 4:14)** Some four years earlier, Hope had been brought to her knees by painful memories, intense conviction, and deep longing as she struggled to pray for a church member who had been diagnosed with cancer. Hope had been at the hospital, preparing to pray for this stricken individual, when she was overwhelmed with images of her own father's death. She was overwhelmed by the sights, sounds, and smells of that remembered time. She became spiritually incapacitated by the present reality of her "faith deficit" against such an invincible enemy. God had chosen this time to speak to her in the strongest, most loving terms possible, about her deep wounds. Even prior to this traumatic moment at the hospital, God had been preparing Hope for an enormous challenge to her faith for the healing of cancer. For example, He would lead her through a spiritual "game of dare" (as she described it) by asking her if she had healing faith for a series of relatively minor ailments: "Hope, do you have healing faith for arthritis, flu, tennis elbow, etc. etc. ?" Hope would "play along" by answering, "Yes, Lord."

This "game" would progress steadily toward the ultimate sickness that had terrified her for so long, when God would ask her, "Hope, do you have healing faith for cancer?" This was the question for which she always came up wanting. At that moment,God told Hope that He was disturbed that so many of His children had lost much of their deepest faith by **"bowing to the idol of cancer,"** accepting defeat and death, time and time again. God had further told Hope that **He was "jealous" and "angry"** that His children had begun to wonder if He was truly sovereign over this disease. He then comforted Hope by telling her that He had been waiting for these many years since her own father's death — waiting to heal her of this wound if she also wished it — for **Hope was also an unwilling slave to the cancer idol**. God wanted to heal her so that she could pray with faith for cancer victims. God desired that His sovereignty and power over all things would be demonstrated to His fearful people. Hope held this incredible "word" in her heart and waited.

Some six months later, as a confirmation for this new, inner healing message, God had positioned Hope as an intercessor for a woman who she thought was having marital difficulties. At the time, Hope was unaware that the woman was actually suffering from cancer of the uterus. It was a condition that the woman attempted, unsuccessfully, to tell Hope about during one very emotional, spirit-filled prayer session. It wasn't until two months after that session that the woman informed Hope that she had received a miraculous healing of her cancer. Tearfully, Hope told me that without these incredible experiences, and God's words of healing to her, she could not have agreed to pray with me, in faith, for my healing. She felt that she was being called, now, to do just that.

As I hung up the phone from this conversation, I was literally overwhelmed by a powerful tidal wave of thoughts, images, feelings, and memories that seemed too spontaneous and connected to be completely natural or even voluntary.

- I remembered my exact thoughts and feelings upon learning of my own father's cancer diagnosis, and how automatically and completely I had given over to the inevitability of his death. I recalled how the period of his treatment had merely represented a preparation, a waiting time, for cancer to take its deadly course. He himself spent much of this same period of treatment preparing for death. His doctor's final prognosis of "six weeks to live" resulted in an almost clockwork-like rendezvous with that death schedule.

- I remembered my family doctor's first emotional words when he first suspected cancer in me ("Oh no, Oh hell, Oh no..."). I remembered how his face had looked. It was as if he was, unconsciously, identifying something deeper and evil about the disease.

- From my past, I recalled the general reaction of most people I had known (including myself) when informed of someone's cancer diagnosis (same horror, same resignation), or a cancer death (no surprise).

- I thought about my reaction to the surgeon's sober, workmanlike expression of cancer's probabilities. The facts had not only informed me, but had quietly disheartened me with a subtle but powerful authority over my mind and my spirit.

- The power of the Internet to create an information explosion of coldly devastating cancer statistics had driven me (and how many others?) to deep despair. What an incredible, modern weapon of spiritual discouragement, disguised as electronic-age enlightenment.

- Hope had described a hidden, spiritual paralysis that underscored the many statements of acceptance and rationalization about cancer == statements that I had heard and even spoken, myself, over the years. "I guess his death is just God's will." "What a blessing that her suffering is over." "God's ways are just mysterious." "Sometimes God just says 'No.'"

- I thought about the language of cancer: words that are not only unique, but sound so natural when spoken about cancer. This language contained expressions such as, "terminal," "radical," "dying of,""survivor," "three- and five-year survival rates," "remission," and "recurrent."

- I thought about my local cancer clinic and all the dedicated cancer clinics and hospitals in every city, in every country, around the world. How special and pervasive this disease had become in order to create a completely separate, institutional system to house it. It was a massive, worldwide system, with its own unique facilities, personnel, and treatment. And, how revered and respected such institutions were; impressive monuments to mankind's battle against the disease.

- I thought about my ongoing struggle with despair, which seemed to be in some kind of "overdrive" mode.

Even as I was recovering from this torrent of thoughts, the decisive blow was struck, sending me reeling even more. The vivid memory of **Isaiah 41:21-24,** with its imagery of the priests of **the idol** (Baal worshippers), predicting the future like gods, sowing fear and disma, suddenly merged into God's words to my friend Hope. This union of memory and experience produced a sort of revelation in my mind and spirit. **It was a realization of an incredible connection between my "coincidental" open Bible reading and a supernatural message that God had first spoken to Hope. A message, which for some reason, He now wanted me to hear**. For the first time in my difficult journey, I had a heightened sense of something taking place beyond my illness.

It was a sense that God was really involved in a manner beyond my mere chastening or punishment. It was too large a coincidence to ignore, even for my jaded sensibilities. And, apart from its "supernatural" origin, this spiritual sense also seemed to make such common sense, as well.

In my experience with cancer, past and present, first as an observer and now as a victim (I so hate that word), I could see that I had been extraordinarily conditioned to assume a unique posture of death. It could be a courageous, even resistant posture, yet ultimately it had to be realistic. I could understand how cancer physicians were in some way set apart, even from the already revered, regular practitioners of medicine. It's often been asserted that we assign almost godlike status to our doctors. It is clear that our extraordinary fear and awe of cancer is often reflected in an extraordinary fear and awe of cancer doctors. This reverence for our physicians is to the point where their prognostic statements have become almost like inerrant "prophecy" to generations of desperate, hope-hungry, cancer patients. This new spiritual sensitivity challenged me to believe that the Isaiah 41 passage was, in fact, conveying an image of these modern "priests." I could also see how easily, and willingly, I had "bowed to the idol" by internally accepting my bleak prognosis and resigning myself to its power, And then by struggling with a faint hope that these doctors, the technology, or even alternative treatment might somehow grant my only chance at life. **I was most disturbed (and convicted) by the realization that, while I believed God had sovereignly allowed cancer to afflict me, my historical "cancer conditioning" had somewhat robbed me of the ability to believe that He would (or could) heal me.** After all, it was cancer. Just look at the statistics. This struggle with the concept of God's sovereignty reminded me of the nuclear weapons dilemna. These weapons had been invented by mankind, but had quickly transformed into such an inherently destructive force that, once unleashed, **even the inventors could not control it.**

But God was supposed to be omnipotent, sovereign over everything, in complete control; the final authority. God had told Hope that He was disturbed that we had "bowed to the idol of cancer." We had surrendered our faith to the idol and its "priests." This surrender had detracted from, had even substituted for, our faith in the true God. God said that He was "jealous" that His children no longer believed He was truly sovereign, and that He wanted to "heal" Hope of her depleted faith and her fear. I reasoned, wishfully, that He wanted to heal me as well. Even as **"the cancer idol"** imagery was still impressing itself upon me, I started to wonder about the generations of conditioning, the ease with which resignation sets in, and the inherent expectancy of death. The conditioning had become a quiet, dignified, absence of hope, and not just an absence of hope within the victims, but within so many others around them (family, friends, caregivers). This was the subtle, insidious infiltration of our mind and spirit by the power of cancer. Even the strong minded, or the apparent strong-of-faith, seemed to give over. This giving over sometimes occurred reluctantly and fiercely. Often, it took place meekly, almost serenely: like sheep led to slaughter. Was there more than just a symbolic or psychological "idolatry " syndrome at work? Even secular psychologists would support the notion of how "negative thinking" affects the welfare of patients. I began to consider — even believe — that there was something much more supernatural behind the incredible culture of cancer. That night, I wrote the following thoughts in my makeshift "journal":

**"The world bows to the idol of cancer ... Doctors are the new oracles and high priests, and cancer clinics are the new temples ... Is cancer the one disease where God does not have sovereignty? ... Cancer makes us like new**

**human sacrifices on the altar of human effort, knowl-
edge, and treatment that secretly affirms death ... Even
the church has gradually been drawn in as a willing, but
unwitting, participant in this mass delusion of the enemy
... A great gig to get, if you're Satan ..."**

Why I wrote this the way I did, I can't say. But I was excited
in a way I had never experienced before, just as I was fearful
in a way that I had never known.

My faith increased as a result of this remarkable experience, and I began to feel that God was somehow creating
these incredible connections and Biblical relationships to
lead me somewhere. I did not yet understand that the spiritual process, by which He was creating these connections and
relationships, actually represented a fascinating set of clues
to a (possible) **"mystery story." It was a story that was,
simultaneously, being told in my life and in Scripture at
the same moment.** For example:

- My friend's "mighty warrior" e-mail reference was
  connected to Gideon, the mighty warrior (Judges
  6-7).
- The Isaiah 41 "threshing" reference was connected
  to Gideon's threshing.
- Hope's "idol of cancer" reference was connected to
  the Isaiah 41 idol/priest passage.

By creating these connections each time, it was as if God
was confirming that I was "on the right track" with my
wondering. I had never had anything even remotely like
this happen to me, and I remember remarking to Lori that,
"If I wasn't so scared, I would just be incredibly excited."
The belief that this horror I was facing had a deeper, underlying meaning or message, sent from God, raised my hope
to a new level. Yet, I was still very skeptical (still feeling

unworthy and shocked), and so, I was more than curious to see if the experience would continue. I guess I needed more proof. I was clearly no "super believer," and my first, official, post-operative consultation at the cancer clinic was to take place a few days hence. Curiousity was probably not the most accurate way to describe my thoughts about that.

# CHAPTER 8

# "AND IN THIS CORNER ..."

I can remember entering the clinic reception area with Lori, giving my name, and then sitting down to wait. I had a kind of surreal awareness that caused me to be conscious of everyone else in the room, while still being able to stay within myself and my own situation. You take everything in, wondering which people have cancer and which people are fortunate enough just to be companions. You just seem to know that everyone is trying to contribute to the outward calm of the place as they read magazines or sip their coffee. Yet, all the while, we quietly rage inside with the questions, fears, and emotional turmoil of this terror disease. Some people actually looked ill, but most appeared as I must have; healthy and vital on the outside, hiding the creature that was silently destroying us on the inside. You find yourself wondering what kind of cancer they have; whether it is milder or more serious than yours. You wonder what statistical probability for survival they have been given. You conclude that the happier looking ones must have a "better" cancer. There was a tangible sense of heaviness in the clinic, a sort of quiet forboding, a peaceful environment of fear. Even as the staff used their special training to keep a light, businesslike, even healing atmosphere, it wasn't working well. I felt like everyone was doing what I was doing. We were all aware of each other. I would come to experience this acute awareness many more times as I built my life around the clinic over the next three months, and as I was drawn ever deeper into this secret world that everyone knows exists, but really doesn't want to understand.

Lori and I were first ushered into a meeting room where we met the surgeon who had performed the biopsy on my tonsils. Something happened here that really demonstrated the incredible fear and grace that walked beside me, as two powerful companions, on this journey. The fear aspect of this event revolved around the prospect of additional surgery to excise any residual cancer or to prevent further spread. In my early Internet research, I had seen descriptions of head and neck surgical procedures, most of which read like a primer on medieval torture. This particular form of cancer often necessitated the surgical removal of vital, soft tissue structures: the tongue, the larnyx, sections of the throat or jaw, or sections of the neck and shoulder muscles, just to name a few of the possibilities. What the cancer information sites blandly termed "morbidity associated with surgery," was described as potential loss of the ability to speak, swallow, or even breath through normal means. I remember thinking that there was a spiritual significance to how God allowed this particular form of cancer to afflict me. Surgery had the potential to prevent me from engaging in one of the deepest passions of my heart: worshipping Him with my singing voice and with my guitar. I remember thinking that it was no coincidence that cancer surgery could directly destroy both abilities. I remember wondering if that was exactly what God was going to allow. Was He so displeased with my efforts to praise Him that He no longer wanted me to possess the ability? Did He see so much pride and self in my alleged worship (that's another story) that I needed to be silenced?

Why had He apparently blessed me over the last few years with increased musical inspiration and skill, just to bring it to an end now? I had been praying about this fear of losing my physical ability to sing and play guitar. Thinking about that prayer, I sat in front of the surgeon, truly wondering if this meeting was the beginning of the end.

The doctor re-examined the surgical area in my throat, seemed satisfied, and said that treatment should commence as soon as my tonsil area healed sufficiently, which would be within a few more weeks. I was almost afraid to ask, but I had to know. Did he feel that further surgery was advisable? Had he been able to remove the tonsil tumor completely? In the same unnerving, businesslike manner of our first meeting, he quickly explained to me that the removal of my tonsils for biopsy purposes could not be considered "proper cancer surgery." Such proper surgery would entail a much more radical approach. The proper procedure would begin with the splitting of my jaw in half, followed by a deep incision in my tonsil area to remove large amounts of soft tissue. Unfortunately, a consequence of this surgery was "considerable morbidity" in functions like speaking and swallowing (no kidding). I was bracing myself for the bombshell, when he followed this by saying, "Because of this possibility for extensive morbidity, in your case I really feel that treatment with radiation alone is the best approach for now. This particular type of tonsil tumour appears to respond quite well to radiation." In shock, I responded, "So you don't feel surgery will dramatically improve my situation?" He replied pointedly, "I've had patients who have **insisted** that I perform the surgery, even with the resulting morbidity, and in my experience, **it doesn't make a lot of difference to the outcome**" (Isaiah 41 again…"say anything good or bad, so that we may be filled with fear"). He continued, "Besides, I think that you have an advanced cancer, and it's important that we don't waste any more time starting treatment" (Isaiah 41 again…).

"We'll see about surgery after your radiation treatment is completed. One step at a time." Inside the shock, the fear, and even the relief that I was feeling, a faint whisper of hope reminded me that I had just been spared (so far) from disfiguring, song-stealing surgery. I was too burdened to decide if it was the grace of God or not.

Lori and I were sent to another examination room where we sat and waited again among the anatomy diagrams and instruments. Finally, the door opened and we met another specialist, a radiation oncologist, accompanied by a nurse and a resident. After some poking and prodding, the doctor proceeded to explain that my cancer was quite serious, having moved already to my lymph nodes, and that he had scheduled me for 35 radiation sessions over a period of two months. He was also recommending that I undergo a couple of four-day chemotherapy sessions during my radiation treatment. There had been recent evidence of complementary, improved results by combining the two therapies. So, chemotherapy too. What next? The oncologist and company were pleasant and reserved, but that only succeeded in increasing the unreal, spiritual burden that had settled on us when we walked into the waiting room. We discussed the basic aspects of radiation therapy, preparatory procedures (further CT scans, casting of an immobilization face mask...What was that?), and, of course, side effects. The side effects were talked about in an almost casual way: mouth dryness, taste changes, skin irritation or burning, tissue weakening, fatigue, possible weight loss. But, there would be counsel and support to deal with the side effects. I was struck by the necessity to deal with the accompanying new illnesses caused by my illness. The friend of my enemy is also my enemy.

Next we found ourselves in another meeting room, with another member of the clinical team: the dietitian. She possessed the same pleasant, forced demeanor that we had encountered so far. We listened as she calmly mapped out my nutritional destiny over the next few months.

- Step 1: Bulk up, eat as much as you can over the next month or so, to gain your maximum weight. Weight loss is the number one healing obstacle for cancer patients.
- Step 2: Once your throat soreness from radiation reaches a certain point, you will need to obtain nourishment from softer food and eventually liquids. So here are some recipes for high protein, high calorie milkshakes. Even with these you will find it difficult and painful to swallow.
- Step 3: If you can't maintain your weight, we may have to admit you to the hospital to be fed by tube. Some patients require this. I made the mistake of acting somewhat confident by saying, "Well, I just had a tonsillectomy, and with the help of pain killers, I seem to be able to swallow OK." Almost as if the rebuttal was ready ahead of time, the dietitian brought me back to reality: "Oh, your throat will be much more sore than it was from a tonsillectomy" (after all, Fred, it is cancer...). I stood corrected.

As we finished this uplifting session, our last visitor, the clinic psychologist, popped in. Not surprisingly reserved and pleasant, he explained that "psychosocial services" were available for all patients who would like to have some help or counsel for coping with the disease and treatment. He was obviously busy, so he left me with a copy of a profile/survey (I would eventually complete it three to four times throughout treatment), which was designed to establish and track my emotional and mental state. I confess that, from the beginning, I did not give this particular aspect of the treatment much attention, as I had decided that my situation was more spiritual at its foundation. Perhaps I sensed that my chances for life were lessened if I counted on my emotional and mental resources for protection or guidance. The psychologist was our last meeting for this first time at the clinic, thank God. At least for that day, I knew that I had been, emotionally and mentally, beaten into submission. Round 1 had gone to cancer.

We left the cancer clinic with this string of consultations playing like a sad movie in our heads. I was dejected and disheartened at the sheer reality of what I was facing for the next few months. The monumental power of cancer, even in the face of our formidable medical and technical arsenal, was shattering to me. These discussions also gave me a more complete impression of the subtle power of the disease over the very people who were responsible to treat it. I can remember imagining these dedicated, sincere people fighting an invincible, maneating monster, themselves poorly armed with primitive sticks and rocks.

**The most significant aspect of this day was coming face-to-face with the power of the spoken word.** Each time the words "serious," "advanced," "morbidity," and "potential spread" were spoken, they seemed to contain an inner force far beyond their clinical meaning. There was a kind of deadly irony to these discussions. We had spoken with numerous physicians who were pledged to administer healing, yet the actual dialogue seemed to be completely bereft of healing words. I could understand the need to be realistic, but there seemed to be a weird sense of detachment in this atmosphere of realism. This detachment increased the emotional and spiritual momentum I was experiencing, and it was a negative momentum. I understood that they were being honest, with the best of intentions, and had no wish to add to my anxiety. Yet, the power behind their realistic words seemed purposeful, terrifying, and deeply spiritual. The words had cut very deeply into my soul.

# CHAPTER 9

# "GET YOURSELF READY"

That evening, as I reflected and prayed about the events of the day, I was gradually overwhelmed by the disheartening reality of my situation. I began to imagine the dreaded cancer cells growing and multiplying inside me, overflowing their original sites in my neck and spreading like locusts throughout my body. I pictured the disease creating new tumors in untreatable places, consuming me from the inside, and finally killing me, slowly and horribly, just as I had seen them kill my father and so many others. I remember trembling as these images spilled over me, while at the same time realizing that I was just at the beginning of this trial. How could I possibly function for the next days, let alone next months, with this overwhelming fear gripping me? In desperation, **I silently cried out to God.** I cried out for a sign, or a word of assurance, to help me deal with the dark abyss I was staring at and was coming dangerously close to falling into.

I turned over the pages of my Bible to begin some of my open reading, and I noticed that I had stumbled into the book of **Jeremiah**. I thought, "Great. Jeremiah is one of those books with all kinds of scriptures about wrath and judgement." But my eyes were immediately drawn to some words that seemed to shout out to me from the first page I looked at.

**"Get yourself ready ! Stand up and say to them whatever I command you. Do not be terrified by them, or I will terrify you before them. Today I have made you a fortified city, an iron pillar, and a bronze wall to stand against the whole land —against the kings of Judah, its officials, its priests and the people of the land. They will fight against you but will not overcome you, for I am with you and will rescue you," declares the Lord (Jeremiah 1:17-19).**

My immediate reaction was inexplicable at the time (although not now) except to say that **I felt as if I was being spoken to directly**, and loudly, somewhere deep in my heart. Not only was I being spoken to, but I was experiencing a spiritual image of God actually holding me by my shoulders and shaking me vigorously, almost as if to bring me out of some hysterical nightmare *(Note: My dad and mom used to do this to me when I had childhood nightmares…hmmm)*. The only thing God didn't do was slap me in the face to "snap me out of it." At the same time, the words of the text seemed to be yielding a deeper meaning to me, just like Isaiah 30 and 41 had, again without any effort on my part.

- **"Get yourself ready! Stand up and say to them whatever I command you" (Jeremiah 1:17a).** This hit me like a "wake-up call" from Someone who knew that I was weakening, and needed to look to someone stronger for guidance and leadership (I remembered speaking words just like this as a secular business leader).
- **"Do not be terrified by them, or I will terrify you before them" (Jeremiah 1:17b).** The truth inside

this command was like "drawing a line in the sand" in my battle with fear. I felt God was saying, "Fred, if you cannot obey me with courage in this critical battle, I will have to give you over to an intensity of fear that you have never experienced and that you may not survive." It was like a moment of truth in a soldier's "baptism of fire" on the battlefield.

- **"Today I have made you a fortified city, an iron pillar, and a bronze wall to stand against the whole land"( Jeremiah 1:18a).** It was as if God knew about the terrifying images of cancer cells breaking through my natural defenses, spreading throughout my body. Was He saying that, from this moment, the cancer in my body would be contained or kept at bay, supernaturally?

- **"... against the kings of Judah, its officials, its priests" (Jeremiah 1:18b).** Who did these people represent? For some reason, I suspected that they were idol worshippers, and guess what? They were. (I checked in the Bible's text notes.) **The connection to Isaiah 41 and the priests of the idol was another clue in the chain that God seemed to be constructing to keep me on the right track.** Did this verse mean that I could supernaturally "stand against" the "realistic" words and predictions of my doctors and believe for a different outcome?

- **"They will fight against you but will not overcome you, for I am with you and will rescue you," declares the Lord"(Jeremiah 1:19).** Was God promising me directly that He would protect and heal me?

Ever since the first Scripture experiences began, I had been considering the possibility that the circumstances of discovery ( my open Bible reading), and the strange connections between seemingly random passages, actually represented a mild form of *rhema* that had been described by Sandra Kennedy. But, I was now forced to confront the excitement (and apprehension) arising in my heart at the thought that Jeremiah 1:17-19 had been delivered as **a direct, personal *rhema* word, spoken to me through Scripture, by God himself.** This was especially because "the word" had been delivered as a direct response to my crying out in fear, and specifically, my fear of the disease spreading. The notion of "pure coincidence" was starting to look like a paper-thin veil that was inadequately trying to cover the light that was starting to pour into my situation. Still, I was fighting a disbelief born of questioning why He would *want* to speak to me this way, and why He would want to speak to one such as me. And, of course, I struggled with the question of my own ability to deceive myself into *imagining* that He was speaking to me, because I so much desired hope. It all seemed so crazy.

I think it's appropriate to mention, again, that although I (allegedly) was a "believer" of relatively long standing, with decent, general Bible knowledge, I was by no means a Bible scholar. I know that a cynical reader of this book might suspect that I somehow consciously selected and pieced together these scriptures to coincide with the non-Bible experiences (the "voices;" Hope's word from God) that I had encountered so far. Although I'm quite aware that people have been known to fabricate "messages from God," it's illogical that I would knowingly *do this to myself*, especially in the matter of my own, very real, life-and-death situation. To the cynics I can only say that it took me a good long time to even acknowledge that these events *might* be supernatural (I'm still kind of reeling from it all). In other words, *I* was probably the *most* cynical and skeptical about these "words from God." I did not really understand the contents of Isaiah or Jeremiah, other than their status as prophetic books. I had always avoided them, in actual fact. Later on, I would be led to many other parts of the Bible that I had not read before, let alone studied or understood. As God continued to pursue me in this way, linking scripture after scripture together in a chain of faith, I finally had to acknowledge that it was, most certainly, not just a string of coincidences. Hopefully, you will grow in belief as the story continues to unfold. I did.

During the next couple of days, I pondered the impact of the Jeremiah 1:17-19 passage on my attitude and outlook for the next steps of my journey. I continued praying, open Bible reading, as well as reading other books by Christian authors. *(Note: Throughout the next few months, I would regularly travel to the local Christian bookstore and browse the shelves for books that might edify and assist me in understanding what was happening in my life. I would select a wide variety of books on prayer, healing, biographies, spiritual growth, the Holy Spirit, spiritual warfare, and general interest. I would read some forty books over the course of three months, and I would receive timely ministry from almost all of them. It was as if I had been led or directed to choose the very books that God wanted me to read. I'll be citing some powerful examples as we progress through the story.)* Although the scriptures I "fell upon," during this time lacked the awesome drama of Jeremiah 1:17-19, my heart responded to the words with a feeling that a kind of foundation was being laid for me. The readings provided some further clues as to how I might better understand my spiritual interaction with what was happening to me. I didn't, automatically, think of the following Bible readings as direct *rhema* words. But, I was to come to an understanding, later on, of how they formed part of the general *rhema* landscape of my journey.

- **Psalm 51:3-4** captured much of the sense of responsibility I was feeling for my dilemma. *(Did I mention before that I never once questioned why God allowed* *me to be afflicted? If I was being chastened, or even punished, I knew that I deserved it more than most.)* **For I know my transgressions, and my sin is always before me. Against you, you only, have I sinned and done what is evil in your sight, so that you are proved right when you speak and justified when you judge.**

- **Psalm 51:16-17: You do not delight in sacrifice, or I would bring it; you do not take pleasure in burnt offerings. The sacrifices of God are a broken spirit; a broken and contrite heart, O God, you will not despise.** This passage helped me understand why He was literally tearing me down, piece by piece, bodily, emotionally, and spiritually. I could see why my previous life of serving Him on the outside, while only being partially committed on the inside, would no longer "work" to curry His favor. It also gave me hope that perhaps I might eventually approach Him more authentically: with a heart He wouldn't "despise." The only problem was, I had no way of knowing when the tearing down would be complete enough to satisfy Him.

- **Psalm 41:5-9** read like a commentary on the faith crisis experienced by many people who gather around someone confronting cancer. **My enemies say of me in malice, "When will he die and his name perish." Whenever one comes to see me, he speaks falsely, while his heart gathers slander; then he goes out and spreads it abroad. All my enemies whisper together against me; they imagine the worst for me, saying, "A vile disease has beset him; he will never get up from the place where he lies." Even my close friend, whom I trusted, he who shared my bread, has lifted up his heel against me.** The word "enemies" might be substituted by the phrase "well meaning but defeated friends and family." It made me more sure of the decision we had made to keep our circle of confidence and prayer a very small group of people. As harsh as the language of this Psalm is, the picture I received was of people who would say openly that they would be praying for healing, all the while not really believing it would (or even could) take place. Or, there was yet another image of those who might visit a cancer victim giving words of encouragement and victory, yet whispering to everyone else on the outside about the imminent defeat and death of the victim. This is no one's fault. I myself had been one of those people.

**Matthew 21:18-22 and 1 Corinthians 13:2b** were examples of the mysterious connections I was shown through various people and media.

- **Matthew 21:18-22** was a scripture I first noted as I started reading accounts of Jesus' healing ministry. Although it is not strictly considered a healing scripture, it is one of the definitive faith scriptures in the New Testament. **It describes the occasion of Jesus cursing the fig tree and causing it to wither so that it would never bear fruit again. He uses the occasion to explain, to the amazed disciples, the principle of "moving mountains:" receiving what we ask for in prayer if we "have faith and do not doubt."** I'm sure that many sick believers have read this scripture, been challenged, and have often been discouraged by it. "Believing and not doubting" sounds much easier than it is. Nevertheless, I read and re-read this scripture, wondering why I had chosen it from the many I had notated earlier. I didn't know that an answer to this question would be provided soon.

- At the same time, I was reading **Father Francis MacNutt's famous book on divine healing called** *Healing*(**Ave Maria Press, c.1999**). In the book he quotes another famous scripture on **the importance of love**, which is **1 Corinthians 13:2b.** This scripture connected itself dramatically to the Matthew 21 scripture, and partially explained to me how having faith to overcome doubt was more within my reach as a result of God's relentless "tearing down" of my heart. The scripture reads, **"… if I have a faith that can move mountains (refers to Matthew 21), but have not love, I am nothing."** I didn't think that Paul had completed Jesus' thought for Him, but merely amplified Jesus' intended meaning. In my case, I wondered if bitterness and resentment, long embedded inside my own heart, had to be **first transformed into love** before I could exercise the faith to believe that my "mountain" of cancer could be moved. MacNutt (along with most teachers of faith and healing) firmly asserts that the absence of a loving heart, or the presence of a bitter heart, could significantly "block" God's healing power, so I know that I am saying nothing new or revolutionary. **It was just interesting that the Matthew 21 - MacNutt - 1 Corinthians 13 connection seemed to happen in an "orchestrated" kind of manner.**

Even though I was pretty sure God had done the "conducting" yet again, I knew that I currently possessed neither the love nor the faith to move any mountains. I also discovered, about a week later, another faith-building reason God wanted me to specifically read Matthew 21:18-22. But for now, these four scripture experiences were, very quietly, "thickening the plot" of the story.

One of the more discouraging aspects of my particular brand of cancer was that even if the primary tumor is treated successfully, recurrence of the disease in other parts of the body is quite common (fifty percent recurrence rate), and most of the time is fatal. For this particular gem of knowledge, I can thank my dogged determination, early in my diagnosis, to research the all-seeing, all-knowing Internet for answers. During one evening where I was struggling particularly hard with this fearful vision of recurrence, I decided to re-read some of the scriptures that I had previously discovered. My plan was to "reinforce" the still fragile hope I had received from those initial readings.

**When I reached the story of Gideon in Judges 6 and 7, I realized that Gideon's story actually extended beyond these chapters into chapter 8, a chapter which I had never read**. Now, you will recall that one of the key, spiritual "mind pictures" I had received while reading about Gideon was the image of the Midianite attack as being representative of cancer in all its invasive and destructive power. I was reluctant to completely adopt the idea that the story of Gideon was somehow, divinely, becoming my story too. However, I couldn't escape the fact that the term "mighty warrior" had been spoken about **both** of us, and that we had both been identified as "threshers" (remember Isaiah 41?). Now, from reading Judges 6 and 7, I knew that the Midianites had been defeated, and if the parallel was truly supernatural, this gave me hope that my cancer would also be defeated. It didn't really occur to me, at the time, that the parallel might extend to the question of recurrent cancer. Although, in retrospect, it would have been logical to assume that many biblical enemies did return from time to time. So I read on until I reached **Judges 8:28-32,** with the unnerving heading **"Gideon's Death"** at the beginning of that section. I remember thinking, "Ok, here it comes, maybe I don't want this to be as much of a parallel." I mean, it was only a few verses removed from the account of Midian's actual defeat. I guess I just didn't understand "Bible time." I read **verse 28: "Thus Midian was subdued before the Israelites and <u>did not raise its head again</u>. During Gideon's lifetime, the land enjoyed peace forty years."** Then **verse 32** read, **"Gideon died at a good old age..."**

My heart was stunned with the prospect that this story really was tied to my situation, and that God was actually speaking to my fear of recurrent disease. I sensed that He was telling me that a defeated cancer enemy would not "raise its head again," and that I would live to a "good old age," whatever that was. It was as if He had deliberately waited to unveil this part of Gideon's story, three weeks after my first reading, and only when the question of disease recurrence was firmly, and fearfully, established in my mind. I immediately began to wonder if I would get some kind of future connection or confirmation for "Gideon's Obituary" (that's what I started to call this text).

# CHAPTER 10

# AN EVIL EMPIRE?

The next significant chapter of my story began a few days later as I prepared to return to the cancer clinic for further consultations with a chemical oncologist, a dental assessment (not clear what this was for), and the fitting of my radiation immobilization mask (*really* not clear what this was for, either). Ever since the day of my diagnosis, I had been haunted by the notion that cancer was not like most other diseases on earth. There were many aspects of the disease that seemed to separate it from "the rest of the pack."

For instance:
- the "special" language
- the respectable and widespread institutionalization inside our culture
- the palpable sense of an unseen "something else" inside the walls of the cancer clinic
- the perenially bleak statistics
- the torturous treatments
- the quiet resignation and "realistic" defeatism of victim and caregiver alike
- the relentless, psychological and spiritual "conditioning" of visions, thoughts, and daydreams. (This

conditioning might not terrorize you to death, but it will calmly convince you that it is reasonable and even responsible to prepare for death.)

- the unspoken "veil of inadequacy" that seemed to cover our faith response to the disease. So many believing victims and families had no other explanation for their ordeal other than "it must be God's will:" the ultimate pressure to surrender.

**I had been reading Smith Wigglesworth's book** *Ever Increasing Faith*, marvelling at the deep assurance of God's miracle power that marked his ministry. In the book he recounts several examples of healing miracles involving cancer, but I had another one of those heart-stunning moments when I read these words: **"When I see cancer, I know that it is a living, evil spirit."** Just as in the case of reading Father MacNutt's book, I felt as if the exercise had been orchestrated so that I would read certain passages, or even a certain sentence, acting as a signal or a catalyst to push me further down the road upon which God had placed me. Suddenly, everything that I had observed, felt, sensed in my spirit, heard, and read to this point started to coalesce into a weird, unified image. **It was as if the clinical and cultural realities of cancer had merged with the spiritual insights I had been receiving to reveal a living picture of how the disease existed, simultaneously, astride the temporal and eternal realms.** Again, I knew that a considerable body of Christians believed that all diseases, not just cancer, were sent from the pit of hell. More broadly, most Christians believed that sickness was a consequence of the original "fall of man" into sin in the Garden of Eden. What really stirred my heart, and shocked me at the same time, was the possibility that the disease of cancer was not only "powered" by an evil spirit, but that, throughout the generations, **this evil spirit had infiltrated and established itself inside a worldwide institution.** It had been able to construct an entire temporal system and culture around itself, complete with millions of deluded victims. Many of these victims were first disheartened, and then destroyed, in an organized, even endorsed manner. This was an intoxicating, complex, and wholly disturbing set of thoughts, yet, **I couldn't deny the spontaneous and quite involuntary nature of the insight.** *(NOTE: I had always possessed a mild form of this kind of insight or intuition in my secular, business life, but I had never experienced anything remotely like this; not of this intensity, not over a sustained period of time, and especially not involving matters that I knew very little about (spiritual, medical). Actually, that's not altogether true. At one other time in my life this overwhelming cascade of spiritual thoughts and images occurred, and that was when I received the conviction of the Holy Spirit fifteen years previous. That is another story for another time.)*

The spiritual connection that seemed to affirm these thoughts was the memory of my conversation with Hope regarding the **"idol of cancer." If God had talked to Hope about bowing to such an idol, was it so implausible to believe that the "living, evil spirit" of cancer had been powerful and active in the world as it sought to satisfy its appetite?** I began to reflect on this hidden, evil activity taking place over many generations. If cancer was also a spiritual enemy, then that meant the enemy had:

- created the idol (the illusion of a mere physical disease);
- influenced the development of temples (special clinics and hospitals);
- spawned rituals (unique treatments);
- appointed priests (doctors, technicians);
- sought worshippers (our humanistic, scientific culture);
- hungered for human sacrifices (victims).

87

Had we unknowingly and yet willingly supported the evolution of this idol, believing in mankind's ultimate ability to heal, while slowly choking off access to the powerful, supernatural source of healing in God? **If cancer truly was an evil spirit, it could never be destroyed by man alone.**

**I began to think about this condition of delusion.**

-   The spiritual foundations of the disease are, inadvertantly, left undiscovered through the sincere, temporal efforts of researchers, doctors, and technicians. It's truly important to emphasize the genuine caring and commitment demonstrated by medical and technical staff engaged in the fight against cancer. Even though they strive to heal inside a system that is undermined by spiritual evil, these incredible men and women represent the best aspects of human compassion and effort. The stronghold that they labour inside of may be infiltrated by the enemy, but they are as much victims of the delusion as the rest of humankind.
-   There is just enough progress in research and statistical life expectancy to give the ongoing hope of eventual, complete victory. There is no doubt that some progress is being made in the medical effort to combat cancer. Many cancers are far less lethal, in the short run, than they were twenty years ago, as a result of earlier detection or improved treatments. On the other hand, many cancers are still as deadly as they ever were. Some cancers are increasing in frequency and are occurring in younger age groups than ever before. A larger, absolute percentage of the population is projected to experience cancer in the future due to multiple factors (environment, lifestyle, etc.). Pop question: Are we really winning the war

on cancer, or is the question so complex that we will never really know?

- Cancer is not the primary cause of death in North America (heart disease is, apparently), but it is the primary enslaver, quality of life destroyer, and killer combined. A recent estimate of the number of people "living with cancer" in North America is ten million. Some will die quickly, some more slowly, and some will remain enslaved, frightened, and subjected to the long-term consequences of treatment (drugs, surgical intervention). Some will be in remission for a while and then die of the disease at a later date. Just because people don't die right away doesn't mean that the "monster" is under control.
- There is a natural preoccupation with fighting the physical manifestation of the disease, although modern medicine is evolving slowly to a more holistic model. This holistic model emphasizes the importance of mind, emotions, and even the "human spirit" in combatting all disease. However, there would likely be a severe amount of skepticism, even mockery (not surprising, but biblical) over the assertion that cancer (or any disease) had a spiritual or demonic basis. There would probably be an even greater skepticism over the idea of an idolatrous, spiritual stronghold being operated inside an earthly institution designed to fight the disease.

Though these ideas were clearly flowing into and through me, I had to admit that even I thought the notion was pretty fantastic. Yet, undeniably, the notion was confronting me. I continued to be excited, frightened, and filled with anticipation for further spiritual connections, confirmations, and words. As I reached the next steps in my own treatment, this idea of the foundation of cancer as a "living, evil spirit" continued to reside deep in my heart. I pondered the possibility that this spirit came complete with a real-world domain, disguised inside the revered system and institution built to treat the disease itself.

As I previously mentioned, my next visit to the cancer clinic was to meet with the doctor who would oversee my chemotherapy. I tried to prepare myself for a couple of anticipated shocks. One, to receive more of the same discouraging "realism" which marked cancer consultations, and two, facing the prospect of chemotherapy side effects, notably the loss of my hair. Although I didn't view hair loss with the same dread I'd had about radical surgery, I knew that my vanity could potentially be another subject that God wanted to "teach" me about. He certainly wasn't leaving much of my identity untouched. Initially, I was pleasantly surprised when I first met this new doctor. He had just returned from Germany where he had attended the funeral of an aunt (who had died of cancer, of all things), but he was decidedly upbeat compared to my other doctors. He explained, cheerfully, that the chemo agent he was prescribing had shown promise in creating a synergistic effect with radiation, and that my chances of survival should improve by at least ten percent! (I guess this is a lot, and it seemed like a lot to someone like me, looking for any increased hope.) He went on to say, cheerfully, that it was important that they arrest the disease "the first time around" because a recurrent tumor did not, statistically, respond as well to the same treatment and was almost always fatal. As if he was saving the best for last, he ended by telling me that this particular chemo agent did not result in hair loss, but that it would cause some of the other common side effects (nausea, fatigue, etc.). When he left the room, I sat there perplexed. Did I just hear good news or bad news? It was Isaiah 41 all over again, in a slightly different package. He sounded more upbeat, more assuring, yet the sum total of what he said had left me even more apprehensive than before (**"Say something, whether good or bad, so that we may be dismayed and filled with fear."**). The chemotherapy would increase my chances by only ten percent. Would I have traded my hair for a twenty percent increased chance? I was "so glad" that he had cheerfully reminded me that I did not want to have a recurrent, and fatal, episode of the disease. I hadn't forgotten that the statistics suggested that I still had an "even money" chance of that taking place. I finished that meeting with a new appreciation for the subtlety of the cancer idol in finding different ways to create despair. I also whispered words of gratitude to God, who had been gracious in the matter of my precious hair as He had apparently been, also, in saving me from debilitating surgery. In my gratitude, I was also asking why, again. He would answer me much, much later.

Just as in normal life, new cancer victims face all kinds of surprises. After I met with the chemo doctor, I sat down with a speech and voice pathologist to discuss swallowing. Apparently, the effect of radiation therapy on the throat was not only to make it "much more sore" than a tonsillectomy (remember the dietitian?), but radiation would also impair the ability of the muscles and structures to transport food properly. More simply, I found out that a percentage of neck radiation patients experienced significant degradation of their swallowing functions. Swallowing would also be affected by the extreme mouth dryness caused by dysfunctional salivary glands. The pathologist was going to do a "baseline analysis" of my swallowing function, pre-treatment, and then update it throughout and after completion. If necessary, she would provide instruction for exercises which might help me maintain adequate function. She again mentioned the occasional necessity to hospitalize and tube-feed radiation patients. Was there *any* good news around here? I guessed not.

No one had to remind me to be on my guard for abnormal psychological reactions to my cancer. I was struggling not to "just give in" to the stark reality of my disease, but instead be practical and still hopeful about treatment. I was also fighting hard not to "spiritualize" every event or experience. I had always believed that God was deeply involved in everything, whether by commission or permission. So, if anything, I was –over-compensating for my normal, spiritualistic leaning by being even more cynical about this constant stream of spiritual insights that were so closely tied to my physical journey. I continued to end up at the conclusion that I wasn't **making** these insights happen. **I was receiving them, or being led to them.**

I was wrestling with these very thoughts as I left the clinic and headed for the parking lot. God's timing again. As I crossed the road leading to the parking lot, I encountered two men walking toward me, evidently heading into the clinic. Their facial resemblance suggested they were brothers, but they couldn't have appeared more different. The first man was dressed in blue jeans, a sports team jacket, ball cap and running shoes. He was walking briskly and comfortably across the road. The second man, dressed in a loose jogging suit, was following a short distance behind. He was walking much more slowly, shuffling his feet like an elderly man. As I drew closer to the second man, it was as if the entire scene shifted into slow motion. This brother was obviously the cancer patient. He had lost his hair from chemotherapy, but his head appeared roughly shaven, as opposed to smoothly bald. His pallor was a kind of chalky, deathly pale, and dark circles underlined his sunken eyes. The veins on his face and hands stood out in contrast to his translucent skin. He had lost so much weight that his face, neck, and hands were literally skin covering bone, and his jogging suit hung in folds on the rest of his body. As I passed him in the crosswalk, I looked into his eyes for a moment, and for that moment I was overwhelmed (again) by an instant image of another person from another time. **For an instant, I felt as if I was**

**looking directly into the eyes of a prisoner in the concentration camps of the Nazi Holocaust.** In the past, I had seen numerous photographs of these prisoners, taken by liberating Allied soldiers. I remembered images of the pathetic, emaciated masses lined up behind barbed wire fences, staring vacantly from inside their dead hearts. I recalled other photographs of disfigured corpses lying on the ground, or in mass graves, faces still contorted in incredible torment. Now, this man's face, and these faces of my memory, again merged into a common picture of suffering, fear, torture, defeat, and death. If he had been wearing the concentration camp's striped uniform, he could have been every prisoner in those horrific photographs. As I my eyes locked with his for that brief moment, I saw something in the depth of his being. It was a presence so chilling, that I couldn't stop myself from quietly murmuring, **"Oh my God, it's the same spirit...the same spirit."** Tears came to my eyes as I passed by him, and as I returned to my own reality, I couldn't escape the thought that God had just given me another powerful confirmation of the timeless power of evil. This evil, personified by the Nazi regime, had the ability to infiltrate, delude, and enslave our enlightened, man-centered world. It was almost too much for me to process the other thought I had, which was that through this connected imagery of another historical "empire of evil," God had also started to confirm the existence of the spiritual foundation of the cancer idol.

The next day, the "good times just kept on rollin.'" My next big surprise came at the dental clinic, where I was given the routine, pre-treatment examination. It was explained to me that radiation therapy on the head and neck region had a significant effect on dental health. The salivary glands would be effected, even to the extent of a virtual "shut down." Normal saliva not only helped rinse harmful bacteria and food particles away, but also contained enzymes which helped protect teeth from plaque and decay (I should write dental-care commercials). Hence, the lack of salivary activity would dramatically increase my risk of progressive tooth decay. In addition, radiation therapy would directly affect my body's ability to repair and restore itself, so that any minor decay would potentially (code for certainly) deteriorate into a major dental problem. "And we don't want to have to do any major dental work on you while you're having radical radiation therapy," declared the cheery dentist. Thankfully, my teeth (fillings, root canals, and crowns notwithstanding) were in "relatively good shape," so I was simply fitted for upper and lower silicone mouth guards to wear each night of therapy. I was also given some fluoride gel to squirt inside the mouth guards, every night. In addition, I was told to wear the mouth guards during each radiation therapy session to help minimize radiation "reflection" off my fillings, which could cause additional burning of the soft tissue inside my mouth (yikes). The "good news" part of this nightmare was that they had only been using this fluoride procedure for about five years. Previous to that, the standard dental protocol for all patients receiving my prescribed radiation therapy was **to simply have all their teeth pulled out;** no teeth, no complications. Oh, sorry, the conclusion to the "good news" was that I had been born late enough to, possibly, keep my teeth. *(Note: As I write, I am thinking about the Nazi practice of "harvesting" the gold teeth of the Jewish dead.)*

I went directly from my dental checkup to the radiation floor of the cancer clinic to be fitted for a radiation immobilization mask. This accessory is primarily for covering the face of the radiation patient, as they lay on the treatment table, so that they might fasten the mask to the table to keep the head motionless. A properly immobilized head maximizes the effectiveness of the precisely calibrated radiation beams. The other benefit of the mask is to enable the radiation therapists to apply ink markings on its surface, providing a "target grid" to line up the equipment and to confirm the treatment areas. In the past, these same markings had to be applied using indelible ink directly to the skin of the neck and face, calling undue attention to the patient when outside the clinic. (So, I guess the radiation mask doubled as a "dignity mask" as well.) As I waited in the designated area, I quietly prayed for the presence of God in the clinic. He is probably there all the time, but I had learned very quickly that the spiritual "oppression" I sensed was definitely present **all the time,** and, in fact, seemed to increase with each successive visit. The technician who was to fit me with my mask led me into the "casting room." This was where a plaster cast of my face was to be made, acting as the base form for the actual clear plastic version. My very first impression (no pun intended) as I entered the room, was of the various plaster casts that had already been made that day. These plaster "faces" were sitting on shelves around the room. Involuntarily, I found myself thinking about the "death masks" that, throughout history, had provided a likeness of the deceased for a tomb or monument. More oppression from the enemy. I knew that these plaster casts were all likenesses of real people facing real treatment, just like me, but the inescapable imagery made me feel as if they were already dead (perhaps some were dead). I'm not sure if this was my first real day of "battling back," against the idol, but I remember quietly praying again, as I lay on the table, waiting for the warm, viscous plaster bandages to cover my face: **"Lord, I look to You to make this a "life mask" for me, not a death mask."** The plaster covered my eyes, and I couldn't see anything, as the formless became form.

The mask story does not end here by any means, and as I think back, I'm amazed at the multiple opportunities afforded the idol (or spirit of cancer) to initiate battles (like this mask thing) for cancer victims. These battles must be fought on multiple levels, and many are often lost while inside the cancer stronghold. The demon seems to exploit respected human virtues like perseverance, courage, and determination. Unless these can be translated into true spiritual virtues, supported by God's power, these frequent, multi-level battles against hopelessness become a delightful "war of attrition" for the demon. This war often prolongs the torture, suffering, and disappointment of the victim, until our human reservoirs of strength are empty, and we are finally, inevitably, overrun by a triumphant, evil army. It can be a slow, methodical conditioning for defeat.

The demon's next attack, involving my radiation mask, was packaged very innocently inside a clinical trial being conducted at the time. My radiation doctor had telephoned me to ask me if I would be willing to participate in a trial initiated to test a new mask design. The experimental design would eliminate the need to first make a plaster cast. The plan was to combine the casting and molding of the mask into a single procedure. The process involved a new material that was ideal for both purposes. There was, primarily, a cost-cutting objective to this clinical trial, but I agreed anyway, just trying to be helpful. I returned to the casting room a few days later, where I discovered that the new material was a type of plastic that was very soft and pliable when placed in warm water, But within a few minutes of being removed from the water, the material dried to a very hard and rigid texture, similar to the original clear plastic. This new material was opaque and contained hundreds of tiny holes for breathing, but the holes were not quite large enough or close enough together to see anything outside very well. The effect was a little confining, although I wasn't claustrophobic by nature. I failed to see how participating in this clinical trial could be wrong for me, or how it could be yet another future battle against the power of the idol. How little I knew.

*(Note: I want to share one additional anecdote from my many encounters with the community at the cancer clinic. I had*

been talking with a caregiver about various issues. He was pleasant enough, more real than many I had met so far, and seemed a little troubled. Quietly, I asked him about it. I was surprised when he inadvertantly shared a "spiritual clue" with me. He said, "I also work, part time, in the main hospital complex [attached to the clinic], but I have to come here to the cancer clinic three days a week to do related work. I don't know what it is, but I just feel uncomfortable, in a weird kind of way, whenever I have to be here. I can hardly wait to get back to the regular hospital." It was a polite articulation of a feeling he probably wasn't supposed to communicate to patients. Yet, I had deeply felt the very same thing the first time I set foot in the clinic. I wondered how many other staff members, patients, or caregivers would admit to experiencing the same "weird" discomfort; perhaps none, perhaps many. Perhaps it was a feeling too honest to be politically correct, and too spiritual to be medically correct.)

# CHAPTER 11

# PEOPLE AND PRAYER

I want to tell you, now, about my pastor and my friend, Warren. I had known Warren for three years, after being connected with him, and our church, under very miraculous circumstances. Over this time, we had grown to like and respect each other very much, and we seemed to have an unspoken affinity and understanding for each other in matters of the church, people, and the spirit. More than anything, we had developed a trust for one another that prompted me to ask Warren to be a partner in the journey along with Lori, Hope and Don. He came from a much more conservative church background (Church of Christ) than I did. And, as a result of pastoring the primarily GenX, postmodern-style church which I had been attending, he also came from a polar opposite origin to Hope and Don (Pentecostal), and even Lori (Charismatic Catholic) for that matter. Apart from the "anointing" I felt about our original connection and my deep trust for his heart, Warren had a life history that prompted me to believe that he was meant to be part of my important battle. In recent months, he had been deeply involved with another close friend and associate who had faced cancer. Prior to my own diagnosis, Warren had partially shared this journey with me. He had been a prayer partner and confidante to his other friend and had witnessed many answers to prayer. He had shared a special depth of insight and meaning, walking beside his friend. The friend's journey, so far (I use this term so often), had culminated in a "remission" of the cancer, as well as a deep, spiritual transformation inside the man himself. I also found out that Warren's father had success-fully overcome colon cancer some fifteen years before. In Warren's words, he "couldn't really think of a close, personal relation who had not overcome cancer..." I believed that he was ready to pray in faith with me. Warren's friendship, his regular ministry and prayer times with me, and his Spirit-led listening and input were to become key connectors to God's story inside my life. God was to confirm Warren's role much in the same way as He had confirmed Hope and Don's. The best kind of spiritual confirmation is when the person confirming doesn't know that they are doing it. This was to happen often with Warren, and it was a true blessing.

After two consecutive days of "cancer realism," I was feeling very discouraged and beat up. But, something had changed in my outlook; subtly, minutely, but nonetheless, noticeable to me. I was frightened, but not *as* frightened. I was still doubting the absolute truth of my early spiritual experiences, but the word "coincidence" was no longer an adequate description either. I was reflecting on the incredible (if unbelievable) spiritual dimensions of my journey at least as much as I was concentrating on the clinical and practical dimensions; perhaps more. I was still preoccupied with my own, personal plight, but I had begun to wonder if I was receiving insight for something beyond my own illness. It gave me some extra hope that perhaps God was not finished with me. It raised my spirits to imagine some kind of God-given purpose and future. "But", as the enemy kept whis-pering, "remember it's cancer, Fred. Dream all you want, but don't forget how deadly it really is." These moments invariably drove me to prayer.

Prior to my cancer diagnosis, I'd characterize my prayer life as being somewhat "robotic" in nature and practice. Oh, I would pray faithfully everyday, working the prayer into my daily routine such as during my morning shower, my evening workout; sometimes driving in my car. And, I would pray virtually the same prayer every day, a predetermined list of people and requests that I had undertaken to mention to God each day. I wasn't ever really sure if God had answered these prayers in any kind of a specific way, but the people I prayed for seemed to be doing OK, so I must have thought "so far, so good." To be fair, there had been some really significant prayers answered for our radio program. As I said earlier in the notes, God seemed to be blessing me greatly in a number of ways until I "hit the wall" of cancer. It was then that I began to realize that my prayer life was mostly an empty pattern, a dutiful ritual, a shopping list disguised as reverence.

*(Note: I can relate one way in which my prayer life immediately changed as a result of my "hitting the wall." In those moments when the whisperings of death became too persistent, I got into the habit of immediately speaking resistance to the enemy. The resistance went something like this: "I refuse to take delivery of that vision of death, and I choose to look to God's vision of life for me." I know that it says in the Bible,* **"Resist the devil, and he will flee from you"***[James 4:7], but I was never too sure that my speaking actually caused him to flee, as opposed to being just a gesture to demonstrate a little courage and a little faith. The whisperings have never gone away. Likely they never will. But, in the face of my experiences with God, the whisperings seem to have lost a lot of their power.)*

My recent clinic experiences were starting to sharply define the strange fear/faith realm that I had entered a month earlier. On one level, it seemed like every encounter with the cancer establishment was deeply embedded in a foundation of fear, and the foundation was getting deeper still. On another level, it appeared that I was receiving spiritual instruction (I'm trying to think of a better word) through Scripture, books, and human words. This instruction gave me a new kind of wisdom (I was still so tentative about this), as well as much needed hope for my future battle on the fear level. The atmosphere around my private prayer times had definitely changed. It was strange how having cancer had exposed my previous, wooden prayer life, in order that I would be enabled to pray more authentically about having cancer. It was like the anti-venom made from the venom itself.

There was a particular night, on the heels of my visits to the clinic, which ended up being yet another new connection, **a prayer connection, to the story that God was writing inside my life.** I sat alone in my dimly lit bedroom, trying to open my mind, my heart, and my fear to God. Probably more out of a sense of duty, I started to thank Him for some of the changes in my life that I had already seen as a result of my illness. I'm not even sure if I was really grateful (I still have problems being "grateful" for cancer). Quite suddenly, I was completely overwhelmed — overcome, really — with **the realization of His grace in my life,** as manifested in these ways:

- The new knowledge of my hardened, bitter heart.
- His love displayed for Lori and me by keeping us together "for such a time as this."
- The renewed connection that He had forged between my sisters and me through my illness (another robotic prayer that He was now answering, His way).
- And so much more (personal stuff to me that I cannot share right now)

This "overcoming" was so powerful that I fell face down on the carpet, weeping uncontrollably, pressed down by a "weight" that I had only experienced one other time in my life. Fifteen years before, when afflicted with chronic fatigue syndrome, I was "crushed" under an overwhelming realization of my own sinfulness. **I was to find out, later, that this was the conviction of the Holy Spirit (Psalm 32:4-5): "For day and night your hand was heavy upon me; my strength was sapped as in the heat of summer. Then I acknowledged my sin to you and did not cover up my iniquity. I said, "I will confess my transgressions to the Lord" - and you forgave the guilt of my sin."** As I lay on the floor weeping, I recognized that the Spirit had, once again, descended "heavily" upon me. Only this time, instead of being overcome with my sinfulness (which was still a very current issue in my life), I was overcome with the realization of His grace for me. I was deeply convicted by how He had pursued me and stayed faithful to me, even though my own faithfulness to Him had just been a prideful "skeleton" of real faith. Even now, in the midst of this affliction which He had allowed for His reasons, God was pursuing me with grace, hope, and new knowledge. I wept even more violently as I pondered why. Why? Why?

Later that evening, when I had recovered from this new encounter with the Spirit, I was sitting, a bit spent, doing some more "open Bible reading." As I turned the pages into the **Book of Joel** (another seldom-visited book), my eyes came to rest on the heading **"Rend Your Heart" (Joel 2:12-27).** My own heart kind of jumped, as it was prone to do almost every time I found myself "hearing and seeing" potential *rhema* words. I wondered if this heading was a "command," or if it was God's way of authenticating what had just occurred in my bedroom. Still, I was again curious to see if there would be some confirmation or connection to my situation, the other scriptures, or my other experiences, that would validate the source of **this** word, this time. I read on.

- **"Even now," declares the Lord, "return to me with all your heart, with fasting and weeping and mourning" (Joel 2:12).** I was doing everything as listed, that night, except for the fasting. That would come later, involuntarily.
- **Let the priests, who minister before the Lord, weep between the temple porch and the altar. Let them say, "Spare your people, O Lord. Do not make your inheritance an object of scorn, a byword among the nations. Why should they say among the peoples, 'Where is their God?'" (Joel 2:17).** As I read this passage, I remembered the image of the cancer clinic as the "temple of the idol." A temple where not just Christianity but any spirituality was viewed as a kind of "positive pill" that might enhance the patient's response to "real" treatment. But because of the high failure rate, it was easy to ask the question that, even if God did exist, where was He when healing was desperately needed? I couldn't escape the imagery of the temple and the altar. It was a place where willing victims, under a powerful, delusional hope of "salvation" (cure), submitted to the ritual promises of the idol, becoming "human sacrifices" to its power. Who were these "priests who minister before the Lord" supposed to be? They were seen to be "weeping" and warning the endless parade of victims and caregivers as they ascended the "temple porch" of the cancer establishment, crying out to the "people" before they were, irretrievably, laid upon the sacrificial altar. Did the cry of "Spare your people, O Lord" mean that more victims could be spared **if someone stood at the entrance,** declaring the Lord's

sovereign presence? Weren't believers already doing this? Perhaps we just thought they were.

- **Then the Lord will be jealous for his land and take pity on his people (Joel 2:18).** This was like God's declaration to Hope that He was **"jealous"** because people doubted His sovereignty over cancer. It resounded and pounded in my heart.

- **"I will drive the northern army far from you..." (Joel 2:20a).** The footnotes for this verse identified the northern army to be either Assyria or Babylon, but a faint memory of the story of Gideon sent me back to **Judges 7:1**, where I discovered that the Midian camp (my first image of cancer) was, "coincidentally," located **NORTH** of the Israelite camp. Another northern army.

- **The threshing floors will be filled with grain; the vats will overflow with new wine and oil (Joel 2:24).** "Threshing" seemed to be a recurrent connection to Judges 6 and Isaiah 41.

- **"I will repay you for the years the locusts have eaten ..." (Joel 2:25).** Lori had spontaneously used these words in prayer the evening before. At the time, I had no idea what the Scripture reference was. I knew now.

By the time I had finished processing this scripture, I wasn't sure if I was reading, hearing, seeing, or conversing; perhaps all at the same time. Yet, I still resisted the call to believe (Why is it so difficult?) that God was being so faithful, so real, and so communicative. My excitement, my faith, and my fear were all growing in intensity, simultaneously. This intensity would escalate even more.

# CHAPTER 12

# BY ANY OTHER NAME

A few days later, my open Bible reading landed me inside a scripture that would be a major turning point in my journey. It would be a new doorway into a deeper understanding of my personal situation. I would gain a deeper insight into the disease that was attacking me. I would more clearly sense the gravity of this battle in the spiritual realm. I would learn that the battle had been raging on for thousands of years between God, the enemy, and our "gods" — our idols. I moved through the pages of the Bible and stopped at the introduction to **the Book of Nahum.** I didn't even know there was a Book of Nahum in the Bible. Perhaps it was the name that intrigued me. I don't know why I stopped there, but I started reading the editors' introductory notes on the book. These notes described the book as, essentially, **a prophecy about the fall of Nineveh, the capital of the Assyrian Empire**, which took place around 612 BC. I was about to flip to another section, out of disinterest really, when I experienced another one of those spiritual "pictures" as I read the following words:

"The Assyrians were brutally cruel, their kings often being depicted as gloating over the gruesome punishments inflicted on conquered peoples. They conducted their wars with shocking ferocity, uprooted whole populations as state policy and deported them to other parts of their empire. The leaders of conquered cities were tortured and horribly mutilated before being executed.... The Assyrian king Shalmaneser III boasted of erecting a pyramid of chopped-off heads in front of an enemy's city. Other Assyrian kings stacked corpses like cordwood by the gates of defeated cities...No wonder the dread of Assyria fell on all her neighbours."

Again, my spirit was literally overwhelmed with a sense that these comments were not just describing the horrible atrocities of an ancient civilization. There was, also, a spiritual connection to the torture, mutilation, humiliation, anguish, and defeat that was being experienced by cancer victims. Cancer patients could be seen as "prisoners of war" that would experience all these cruel "punishments"(surgery, treatment, side effects) before being "executed" anyway. Many cancer victims could look forward to being "tortured" mercilessly by the extreme, radical treatments that often made no difference in the ultimate death sentence of the disease. In addition to the images of inhuman cruelty, the references to populations being uprooted and deported as state policy all resonated with some of the **Nazi Holocaust connections** I had sensed. There was so much chilling, spiritual energy flowing in me, just from reading this introduction, that I was almost afraid to read the actual scripture. But I had to read on, just to see if anything inside the text would confirm these vivid, initial impressions.

- I turned the page and started reading: **An oracle concerning Nineveh. The book of the vision of**

**Nahum the Elkoshite. The Lord is a <u>jealous</u> and avenging God ( Nahum 1:1-2).** There was Hope's quotation, again, right up front. God was jealous.

- **The Lord is good, a refuge in times of trouble. He cares for those who trust in Him, but with an overwhelming flood he will make an end of Nineveh; he will pursue his foes into darkness (Nahum 1:7-8).** This sounded like a prediction that I was supposed to hear. In addition to the initial cancer imagery involving Assyria, Nineveh represented the "epicentre" of the quake.

These next passages all followed the words *"This is what the Lord says:"*

- **Whatever they [Nineveh] plot against the Lord he will bring to an end; trouble will not come a second time (Nahum 1:9).**
- **Although I have afflicted you, O Judah, I will afflict you no more (Nahum 1:12).**
- **You [Nineveh] will have no descendants to bear your name (Nahum 1:14).**
- **No more will the wicked invade you [Judah]; they will be completely destroyed (Nahum 1:15).**

Although I read these passages in different places in the book, I was reminded of my fear of **recurrent** cancer. Perhaps I was being told, repeatedly, that, once healed, it would not return. I thought about the portion of Scripture that I had nicknamed "Gideon's Obituary," where it says, "Midian did not raise its head again..."

- **"Now I will break their yoke from your neck and tear your shackles away" (Nahum 1:13).** This passage really personalized Nahum for me. How "coincidental" that my particular disease manifestation was primarily in my neck. I really felt like God was speaking directly to my situation here.

- **"I will destroy the carved images and cast idols that are in the temple of your gods" (Nahum 1:14).** My initial image was of the radiation mask that had been "cast" from my face, which was patiently waiting for me inside the clinic. Later on the meaning of "idol" would expand greatly.

- **"An attacker advances against you, Nineveh. Guard the fortress, watch the road, brace yourselves, marshal all your strength!" (Nahum 2:1) Draw water for the siege, strengthen your defenses! Work the clay, tread the mortar, repair the brickwork!" (Nahum 3:14).** Cancer was clearly a difficult opponent. It would ferociously defend itself, even against the power of God.

- **Where now is the lions' den, the place where they fed their young, where the lion and the lioness went, and the cubs, with nothing to fear? The lion killed enough for his cubs and strangled the prey for his mate, filling his lairs with the kill and his dens with the prey (Nahum 2:11-12).** I immediately saw a picture of the spirit of cancer (the lion) residing deep in the spiritual structure (the den) of the cancer establishment. In turn, he fed and nurtured the other demons (the cubs) that ruled this particular stronghold for him. Between them, they stalked the hallways of cancer clinics, looking for prey to strangle and kill, thus continually "filling his lairs" with the victims.

- **"I am against you," declares the Lord Almighty. "I will burn up your chariots in smoke, and the sword will devour your young lions" (Nahum 2:13).** In this short statement, I saw a message of

God's fierce opposition to cancer, and for the first time, a suggestion of the real key to treating and curing the disease. Conventional treatments would combat ("burn up") the cancer cells or other physical manifestations of the disease. The truth of the Word of God ("the sword") would destroy the "evil life" or spirit which empowers the disease, expelling it forever. This was an early picture of the actual cure.

- **All your fortresses are like <u>fig trees</u> with their first ripe fruit; when they are shaken, <u>the figs fall into the mouth of the eater</u> (Nahum 3:12).** I was amazed at being reconnected to my reading of **Matthew 21:18-22 (Jesus cursing the fig tree).** Was God bringing this imagery back to me so that I would see the cancer the way He saw it? Was cancer something that could be "cursed" with the Word of faith, even to the extent that the "tree" (the tumor?) would wither and its "fruit" (perhaps spreading cancer cells?) would fall into His "mouth" and be consumed? Never to bear evil fruit again?

- **You have increased the number of your merchants till they are more than the stars of the sky, but like locusts they strip the land and then fly away" (Nahum 3:16).** This passage recalled to mind the hundreds of thousands of Internet websites: marketing, promoting, testifying to the latest alternative and even "miracle" cures for cancer. All were available for a price, and most of the time were not covered by health insurance. For the first time, I pondered the possibility that they were also part of the delusion of hope that the cancer idol used to entice, encourage, even financially harm victims. Most of these "promises" brought only disappointment and dashed hopes. This passage suggested that many of these alternative "cures" were a clever part of the demonic stronghold. Many, in fact, have been proven to be cruel hoaxes.

- **Nothing can heal your wound; your injury is fatal [Nineveh]. Everyone who hears the news about you claps his hands at your fall, for who has not felt your endless cruelty? (Nahum 3:19).** Upon reading this I thought, *Oh Lord, may your conquest of cancer come to pass. There is literally no one who hasn't been affected, in some horrible way, by the enormous cruelty, and emotional devastation of this disease.*

The entire body of the Book of Nahum recounts this incredible battle between the fortress of Nineveh and the armies of the Lord. The outcome is never in doubt, even though the Assyrian fortress is seemingly impregnable, and lethal, to ordinary men. It is a doomed, evil empire, crushed under the jealous, sovereign power of God. I had been brought to an incredible Bible destination. It unified many of the experiences and readings I had previously received and, most importantly, convinced me that I was gaining extra insight over and above that of my **own** illness and my own future. It appeared that God, if He was truly speaking to me in this way, was not just trying to assure me of His healing provision for me alone. He was also explaining something of much deeper significance about the nature of cancer itself. So, for the first time, I wondered if these *rhema* words were just for me, or possibly for others as well, for reasons unknown to me. With my heart feeling the pendulum swinging toward hope, here's what the Storyteller had told so far, inside the mysteries of His Word and through a chosen community of believers:

- Jesus' healing ministry is a picture of God's own healing will for all who are sick and broken. If Jesus is God, and if Jesus is the same yesterday, today, and forever, this healing will is meant for us today.

- The only record of Jesus' inability to heal is on the occasion of "amazing" unbelief. So then, **ordinary** believers who have normal faith struggles and doubts shouldn't be deterred from seeking their healing from God.
- God was actually trying to speak to me. He was being very persistent in breaking through my strong cynicism by causing so many seeming coincidences to steadily occur, but there were too many to be merely coincidences. In addition, these coincidences were occurring in a kind of organized sequence and were amazingly connected to each other. They were all relevant and timely to my current circumstances. They combined human, literary, and scriptural experiences, all complementing and confirming one another. (In spite of this, my doubts continued. It was a struggle without end.)
- I was clearly being led to scriptures that carried meaning beyond (or beneath) their obvious and accepted historical or scholarly meaning. I was somewhat troubled by this, as I was reluctant to attach additional, perhaps erroneous (or even heretical?) meaning to any Bible text. *(Note: Later on, I was to find out that this sense of deeper meaning is legitimate and prompted by God. For example, this deeper meaning is often found within the spiritual mechanism of parables, proverbs, or "dark speech" as they are sometimes called.)*

It was difficult to refute the sheer spontaneity and power of the spiritual imagery I was seeing in these scriptures. I tentatively came to the following conclusions, feeling most unworthy, and, mostly in denial:

- God had first identified me as a "mighty warrior" (a la Gideon) for some reason.
- The Midianites (Book of Judges) were my first biblical picture of cancer.
- God had spoken to Hope regarding an "idol of cancer" that had actually placed mankind in a posture of delusional "worship," leading to suffering and death.
- This concept of a "cancer idol" was being confirmed by multiple, scriptural images of priests, oracles, temples, altars, and sacrifices.
- Some respected Christian teachers believe that cancer has a spiritual foundation or component.
- God was trying to encourage me to look to Him and believe for healing, even in the face of discouraging statistics and clinical predictions.
- The promises of healing and protection had appeared in Scripture very early in my journey. These incidents were very timely and personal. These texts seemed to identify me pretty specifically (*rhema*). A more generalized promise (*logos*) would not have produced such a spontaneous witness in my heart.
- My experience with the "holocaust/cancer victim" in the hospital parking lot affirmed my sense of a demonic foundation. But, even further, the experience also suggested an entire spiritual stronghold, institutionalized within the cancer establishment. Even more disturbing and mystical was the spontaneous connection to images of the Nazi holocaust. They were, perhaps, not the same spirits, but certainly kindred.
- The Nahum experience supported the fortress or stronghold imagery. It identified Assyria (Nineveh) as another biblical picture of cancer. It also spoke of God's jealousy and commitment to destroy the enemy stronghold. Was He going to destroy cancer totally? Why hadn't He?

I must admit that, even as I was (evidently) receiving more of this deeper knowledge or insight from Scripture, my doubts and defenses seemed to increase as well. I remember remarking to Lori that I was sure that any respectable, believing Christian would be full of joy and supremely confident having received such "revelation." But, I kept on second-guessing the experience. I mean, it still could be an invention or self-delusion of some kind. In hindsight, it was also wholly possible that the enemy was increasing the pressure to disbelieve and fear, while seeing this incredible story unfold. Spiritual warfare was escalating. Even with my continual second-guessing, I was undeniably captivated by the sheer wonder and mystery of what might be revealed next. I wondered:

- Would God continue to connect the links in the Scriptural and experiential chain?
- Would He continue to confirm the theory of the demonic stronghold and the idolatry that made cancer so distinctive and deadly?
- Was the connection to the Holocaust a valid one?
- If the spiritual theory concerning cancer was true, would He give understanding of why the stronghold was allowed to exist in the first place, and how it grew so powerful?
- How would the question about the devastating power of cancer versus His sovereign, healing will be explained and answered?

A few nights later, my understanding and my amazement would take a giant leap.

*(Note: I should mention here that I was continuing in my preparation for treatment to begin in about two weeks' time. I had attended another appointment at the clinic radiation*

*unit to undergo a "simulation" procedure, utilizing my newly cast radiation mask, to ensure that the real radiation beams would find their true mark. The procedure involves lying in the CT scanner while wearing the mask, as a technician takes a felt marker and draws crosses and symbols on the mask. These symbols coincide with laser target points to be used for lining up the radiation equipment for each treatment. I was not to personally escape the infamous felt marker, as the technician had to draw a black line on my chest [which would have to stay there and be "touched up" from time to time] for the same targeting purpose. I also experienced, for the first time, the mask itself having to be snugly clamped down over my face with threaded bolts. You will recall that I had agreed to participate in the clinical trial involving the new "one step" mask material. You will also remember that this mask was virtually opaque plastic, except for tiny pinholes meant for breathing, and with no eyeholes. I remember feeling somewhat claustrophobic, which is rare for me, as I lay under this tightly clamped mask for some fifteen minutes as the technician got everything just right. It was a relief of sorts to find out that the actual radiation treatments would normally take only five minutes or so. Still, the experience left a subtle impression, for the future, upon my heart, as well as a definite impression on my face. The pressure of the mask had imprinted a deep, waffle-like pattern in the skin of my face that took a couple of hours to go away (another pleasant little surprise from the idol).*

# CHAPTER 13

# THE 50% SOLUTION

A couple of days later, I was engaged in another open Bible reading session, and I casually turned the pages into the **Book of Isaiah** again. Not long after, my eyes came to rest on the heading **"Israel the Chosen"** (Isaiah 44:1).

- As I read the words, **But now listen, O Jacob, my servant, Israel, whom I have chosen. This is what the Lord says ... "Do not be afraid, O Jacob, my servant, Jeshurun [upright], whom I have chosen"** **(Isaiah 44:1-2).** I remembered the emotions I had felt earlier in the journey while reading Isaiah 41, which spoke of Jacob being chosen as well. I wasn't so full of myself to believe that I had been "chosen" like Jacob, but perhaps God used the thought to encourage me to be brave and to listen to His instruction.

As if verse 1 was the doorway to the hallway to the **real** doorway, I was brought to the heading **"The Lord, Not Idols"** (Isaiah 44:6). I read on.

- **Do not tremble, do not be afraid. Did I not proclaim this and foretell it long ago? You are my witnesses. Is there any God besides me? No, there is no other Rock; I know not one. All who make idols are nothing, and the things they treasure are worthless. Those who would speak up for them are blind; they are ignorant, to their own shame (Isaiah 44:8-9).** God was evidently setting down the distinction between His truth and the lies of an idol. It was quite possible for us to be deluded and unaware of our error (blind, ignorant) as we believe the idol's promises. We could understand, too late, that such belief was "worthless." As a cancer patient, you experience, very early, the temptation (and the pressure) to place all of your hopes in the power of the cancer establishment.

- **Who shapes a god and casts an idol, which can profit him nothing? He and his kind will be put to shame; craftsmen are nothing but men. Let them all come together and take their stand (Isaiah 44:10-11).** All I could think of when I read this passage was my own mask-casting sessions, in which the original technician had to call in two more helpers to assist him in the procedure. They too, had "come together," and gathered around me to "shape" and "cast."

- **The carpenter measures with a line and makes an outline with a marker; he roughs it out with chisels and marks it with compasses. He shapes it in the form of man...that it may dwell in a shrine (Isaiah 44:13).** As if on cue, the text seemed to be speaking about my recent CT simulation procedure. I pictured the calibrations ("compasses") drawn on the mask, and the felt "marker outlines." Later on, as I saw many of these masks lined up on shelves in the treatment rooms, I was reminded of how they, too, "dwelt in the shrine" of the idol.

These scriptures brought me into an intensely emotional place with God. It was a kind of crying out, an acknowledgment that I was finally "getting it." It was as if my darkened heart was finally responding to His communication *with* me and *to* me. These Bible scriptures had been read by millions of people throughout history, yet by supernatural grace, these same words were describing **me**, in **my** time, in **my** circumstances with incredible accuracy. God used this intense, personal realization to open my spirit even further to the knowledge contained in the very next section of the text.

- **He [man] cut down cedars, or perhaps took a cypress or oak. He let it grow among the trees of the forest, or planted a pine, and the rain made it grow. It is man's fuel for burning; some of it he takes and warms himself, he kindles a fire and bakes bread. But he also fashions a god and worships it; he makes an idol and bows down to it (Isaiah 44:14-15).** From this passage I had a picture of mankind's sincere effort to treat and cure cancer. He pursued knowledge, conducted research, and had discovered some effective, practical treatments for the disease ("fuel for burning," "warms himself," "kindles a fire," "bakes bread"). But through this process, man had somehow persuaded himself that he was self-dependent, and that it was just a matter of time until total victory (complete cure) was achieved. He had convinced himself that treating the disease **his** way was the complete way, the right way, the only way, **the sacred way**. Only a part of the man-made solution was true; the rest of the hope was a delusion, "an idol." That's why there were so many partial cures and so many lives not lived to completion. The other part of the man-made solution to cancer was merely an idol nurtured by our faith in man. And, we had begun to bow down and worship it as if it were a god.

- **Half of the wood he burns in the fire; over it he prepares his meal, he roasts his meat and eats his fill. He also warms himself and says, "Ah! I am warm; I see the fire." From the rest [the other half] he makes a god, his idol; he bows down to it and worships. He prays to it and says, "Save me; you are my god" (Isaiah 44:16-17).** The word "half" in verse 16, and my memories of the cancer statistic of a 50 % survival rate, exploded in my spirit. Fifty percent equals half. All I could manage to think, in the midst of this explosion, was, "No wonder 50% is the deadly truth about cancer. **Man has lost the other 50% of the cure to idolatry!** We become lost through believing and worshipping the cancer "idol." How could man hope to cure a physical disease that had an evil, spiritual power behind it? Yet, how often did we "pray" to the man-made "gods" of treatment? We did "pray to the idol." We cried to the cancer-treatment idol, "Save me; you are my god." The "god" often didn't deliver us.

- **They [man] know nothing, they understand nothing; their eyes are plastered over so they cannot see (my eyes were literally plastered over while casting the mask), and their minds closed so they cannot understand (Isaiah 44:18).** The pervasive power of the idol keeps us in a quiet, fearful state of ignorance. We are mostly unaware of our complete capitulation to the predictions and ministrations of the cancer idol. This is most evident when believers make their obligatory, often feeble, attempts to seek God for a healing that they secretly believe will never come. Even such prayers are a signature of the idol's power.

- **No one stops to think, no one has the knowledge or understanding to say, Half of it I used for fuel; I even bake bread over its coals, I roasted meat and I ate. Shall I make a detestable thing from what is left? Shall I bow down to a block of wood? He feeds on ashes, a deluded heart misleads him; He cannot save himself, or say, "Is this thing in my right hand a lie?"** (Isaiah 44:19-20) I was almost spent, emotionally, as I read this passage. "No one stops to think, no one has the knowledge or understanding…" This wasn't meant to be some kind of "lightning bolt" supernatural light show. This was meant to be a dose of common sense to believers who were really listening. Half measures are being taken against a whole disease; part biological, part spiritual. One half of the cancer solution is man-made and useful, the other half is man-made and "detestable." What is left is just a "block of wood" designed to consume our hope. Because of our "deluded heart," we can never "save" ourselves or recognize that the idol in our "right hand" is a "lie." **And as a result, we will never reach the other 50% of the complete "cure" for cancer that is available from God.**

My shattered sensibilities allowed for one more incredible connection to God's *rhema* strategy for me. From **Isaiah 41:13** (a scripture I had received a month prior) the words **"For I am the Lord, your God, who takes hold of your right hand and says to you, Do not fear; I will help you"** were brought back to my heart. It was an amazing picture of His willingness to take my **"right hand"** in healing, if I could only rid myself of "this thing in my **right hand**" that was a "lie" (Isaiah 44:20). I was being shown that "this thing" was the idol of cancer. **From that time on, I began to think of God as "God of the 100% cure for cancer."**

# CHAPTER 14

# ABRAHAM BELIEVED

As I approached the final week of preparation for my treatments, I received what I can only describe as "seed experiences" for future messages and images that God would eventually be sending to me.

-   In my weekly dialogue and prayer time with Warren, he mentioned to me that he had been studying Abraham as resource material for a thesis he was writing. Warren knew that I was struggling with my faith, even in the face of some of these amazing scriptural insights (all of which I was sharing with him). He said to me, **"You really need to read about Abraham."** Most believers know that his story is one of faith, purpose, and blessing. The Bible references that Warren gave me were **Genesis 12:1-3, and Genesis 15:1-7.** Both passages spoke of God's commission and covenant with Abraham. What was Abraham's response to God? Faith, belief, confidence, and obedience. I will admit the scriptures encouraged me a little, but at the same time, they didn't generate any kind of spontaneous, spiritual fire in my heart. What they did give me was knowledge in waiting.

- The next day, during our weekly prayer time with Hope and Don, Hope told us that she had made contact with a gentleman who had been miraculously healed of a brain tumor. She had heard of his testimony from a mutual friend and had arranged for all of us to meet for lunch in a couple of weeks. We would talk about cancer, healing, and faith. I was hoping that meeting such an individual, who God had apparently healed, would provide some kind of clue or key to the process. In her short conversation with the gentleman's wife, Hope had asked if she could think of any particular thoughts or motivations that might have helped her husband receive his healing. The wife commented that her husband had sensed that God had a burden for some unsaved members of the man's family. There was a sense that perhaps God wanted to preserve her husband's life so that he could be a "spiritual patriarch" to his family. The choice and timing of the term "patriarch" intrigued me (again), and I couldn't help but think (again) about Warren's encouragement to read about Abraham, another patriarch.

A couple of days later, during an open Bible reading session, the pages, more or less, just fell open at **Romans 4.** The heading was **"Abraham Justified by Faith."** My amazement was back. As I read through **Romans 4 and into chapter 5**, in somewhat of a daze, I knew that I was being "spoken to" again. God was speaking to me about my two greatest struggles: my weak faith and my need for hope. The following passages actually increased my struggle at that moment, but were foreshadows of a breakthrough later on.

- **Therefore, the promise comes by faith, so that it may be by grace and may be guaranteed to all of Abraham's offspring – not only to those who are of the law but also to those who are of the faith of Abraham (Romans 4:16).** Was I being "promised" something? Was I being pointed to Abraham's faith example? Impossible standard, I thought. I mean, we're talking about *Abraham* here!

- **Against all hope, Abraham in hope believed and so became the father of many nations, just as it had been said to him (Romans 4:18).** It was so easy to give in to the cancer idol and completely lose hope, as the idol had programmed so many victims throughout the generations to do. But Abraham believed what had been said to him, and so he held on to hope. *If* God was truly speaking to me, was there any reason *not* to believe what He was saying to me?

- **…being fully persuaded that God had power to do what He had promised (Romans 4:21).** I knew that God's power (and sovereignty) over cancer was one of the key issues in the battle with the idol. And unless I believed this first part about His power, then the promised part wouldn't amount to much.

- **Therefore, since we have been justified through faith, we have peace with God through our Lord Jesus Christ, through whom we have gained access by faith into this grace in which we now stand (Romans 5:1-2a).** Could I possess this faith that gained access into this grace, and was also sufficient to receive the promise?

- **…but we also rejoice in our sufferings, because we know that suffering produces perseverance; perseverance, character; and character, hope. And hope does not disappoint us, because God has poured out his love into our hearts by the Holy**

**Spirit, whom he has given us (Romans 5:3-5).** I was suffering, but I wasn't so sure about my perseverance or character. But, Abraham hoped and believed too. If I could achieve that same kind of hope, I would not be disappointed or let down. (*Perhaps impossible,* I thought to myself; *I mean, we're talking about Abraham.*)

In all honesty, neither my faith nor my hope was dramatically transformed by this scripture moment, **but I did know that I was being called to reflect upon Abraham.** The connections from multiple sources pointed to that. Later on, I was to come to a more complete understanding of this experience. At this moment, although I didn't consciously think about it, God was treating me like an infant, feeding on formula. The **"solid food" (1 Corinthians 3:2)** was being saved for later. The true nature of grace, hope (as expectation), faith as a gift from God (not of ourselves), and the work of the Holy Spirit were still somewhat mysterious to me. This understanding would unfold when I truly needed it and was ready to receive it with an open and broken heart. Then I would fully understand why Warren had been prompted to speak of Abraham to me. **And, I would understand why cancer victims, just ordinary believers, can follow Abraham's example as they seek healing**.

(*Note: One of the key issues that I wrestled with throughout this journey was the acceptance, in faith, that these scriptural experiences were indeed personal* rhema *words from God, translated by the Holy Spirit. It is clearly an area of great controversy for believers. I have previously mentioned the well accepted [and correct, I believe] teaching that all Scripture represents a universal message, or* logos *word, applicable to all mankind. Sandra Kennedy cautions those who are seeking healing from God about simply* **"adopting"** *random scrip-*

*tures for themselves [by self-will], or* **"claiming" specific outcomes from God on the basis of general, scriptural statements.** *It bears repeating that Dr. Kennedy stresses a commitment to seeking God's* **specific will** *in prayer and through the reading of Scripture. In this way we can receive a strong, direct, and personal communication of God's will for us. This teaching also establishes that there isn't any kind of "continuity clause" in God's healing covenant. God is not bound to deal with everyone in the same, "cookie cutter" way. Jesus and the apostles facilitated the healing of different individuals in different ways. A good illustration of this principle is found in the various methods that they employed to heal blindness. God provides an individual* rhema *"word of healing" [consistent with His general healing will] through prayer or hearing of the Scriptures.* **This "word" is personal and unique to each believer.** *One of the great gifts of this journey was the conviction that such personal "words of healing" from God are available to many more afflicted believers than is evident today.)*

# CHAPTER 15

# DREAM A LITTLE DREAM

At the beginning of the final week of preparation, before the commencement of my treatment, a brand new realm abruptly intruded into my life: **the realm of dreams.** On a macro level, the debate over dreams is time honored. Dreams have been studied, discussed, and revered by every generation in history. Whether the basis for the evaluation is religious, para-religious, medical, psychological, tribal, pharmaceutical, or cult–based, dreams are considered significant in understanding just who we are. More narrowly examined, the Bible portrays the dream as an important method of communication from God to mankind. On a personal level, I had always dreamt a lot, but almost never really remembered my dreams, even though I believe I possess an above-average memory. I will say that, prior to the dream event that I'm about to relate, I had experienced (and remembered vividly) only a couple of other dreams that I would describe as important and spiritual. The first was a dream just prior to my father's death, some eighteen years before, and the other occurred during my first major, life-changing illness fifteen years prior. You can see why I did not consider dreaming a major, ongoing part of my relationship with God. I was really not expecting to receive any significant "connective activity," via the dream medium, to my other personal and scriptural experiences. **Even as I write these words, I am marveling at the persistent love of God in attacking my doubt and fear on so many levels, and from so many directions.** It's as if He knew just how weak and cynical my faith had become. Yet, He loved me relentlessly, and desired my understanding so much that He went out of His way to present the evidence.

My dream took place inside a large boardroom, elegantly lit, with a large oval conference table in the middle, surrounded by a number of smaller, oval tables. There were several business people sitting around each table (approximately 20-30 people in total). Their features were difficult to make out because of the tasteful, but dim, lighting in the room. I was standing in one corner of the room with my family business partners (my cousins Mike and Mel) and a very trusted senior colleague (Bob). We were obviously there to make a business proposal of some kind, because Mel and Bob were practicing their portion of the program using a power-point presentation on a wall screen. **But I knew that it was my responsibility to make the main sales pitch and to lead the discussion from "our side of the table."** *(Note: I'll briefly mention here that in my many years as a secular businessman, I had been given this responsibility on numerous occasions, and had been blessed to be involved in many of the key, successful presentations which positively changed the course of our business and our financial future. So, the environment portrayed in my dream was a familiar one.)*

As I walked to the head of the large conference table at the center of the room, I can remember feeling the familiar exhilaration, apprehension, and anticipation that had always preceded these moments in my business life. I began the presentation in a confident, professional manner, but I don't remember the details of the presentation itself.

I do remember feeling as if it was flowing along well, and that I had the attention of the entire room. I came to the end of my briefing and asked for questions from the attending group. Suddenly, I was very abruptly engaged by an older (but not elderly) man. He was at the same, large conference table, sitting directly across from me. It was quite obvious that he was the either the senior executive or the CEO of the group. Everyone seemed to be deferring to his leadership as he questioned me. He asked several pointed, but polite, questions about the content of my presentation. After listening patiently to the questions, I replied with thoughtful and complete answers. My responses seemed to increase his interest, but also seemed to increase his aggressiveness in questioning me. It seemed that he was trying to agitate me, to knock me "off-stride," so to speak. But I continued to answer even the most difficult of his questions with patience and certainty, looking straight into his eyes as I responded. The energy level in the room was intense, and it was clear that everyone was focused completely on this important exchange between the CEO and me. In my heart, I just knew that this meeting was critically important to the future of our company and to my own future.

Finally, looking straight at me, the CEO asked, very sharply, "Are you absolutely sure about your case? Are you absolutely sure that your company can do this job?" I looked straight back at him and answered calmly, with a strong voice, "Yes sir, I am." The room was silent. He seemed a little offended and was frowning slightly, deep in thought. I knew enough not to say anymore. The silence seemed to go on forever. Suddenly, he burst out laughing and said something like, "Well, I guess you just told me a thing or two." He said this warmly, with a smile on his face. He then turned to his colleagues and said something that seemed to endorse me to the rest of the group. The tension in the room lifted. I knew this feeling really well. *Everything is going to be*

*OK,* I thought to myself in my dream. We were going to get the contract, even though nothing formally had been spoken about it. Then, just as I was moving away from the table, he turned to me and asked me another question. **"What is your name, again?"** I replied, "Fred." He turned again to his colleagues and spoke some short words of introduction about me. I moved away from the table, and from the corner of my eye I could see my partners making their way to the main conference table for their portion of the program. The last thing I remember is that I just left the conference room, not even bothering to wait for the end of the meeting. I walked away knowing that we had been successful, and that everything was going to be OK.

When I woke up, the memory of this dream was etched in detail on my mind and heart. It reminded me of some of the most blessed times in my life. Times when I had dared to believe in something new and innovative; when I had been confident and wise; calm and forceful; sincere and ethical; compelling and sensitive to others — and, of course, times when I had been healthy. I remembered that it was at these very moments in my secular business life that I had felt God's blessing and His good plans for me and my family. Those times seemed so distant from me right now, but I couldn't deny the deep impression that this dream had left on my heart. But still the doubts ran through my mind: dreams are just wishful thinking while we sleep, right? They are merely imaginings created by our own needs, fears, and desires, right? I knew that I had to investigate this vivid, detailed, remembered dream. I needed to satisfy the stirring in my heart that wouldn't go away.

I decided to go back to the infamous Internet, only this time I searched for sites devoted to Christian interpretation of dreams. Again, I was amazed at the vast number of sites available, and it took me awhile to distill out the sites that were Christian from those that were just "mystical" or "mythical" or "new age." I was finally led to a very straight-forward "checklist" for dream evaluation, managed by a reputable, Christian organization. The checklist outlined five key criteria for determining which of our dreams might be viewed as divinely inspired or sent.

- The memory of the dream would be unusually or uncharacteristically vivid and detailed.
- The self-awareness level inside the dream would be very real. How we felt, how we looked, what we said, what we saw, how we reacted or responded would all be very definite and very familiar. This self-aware-ness would be close to a feeling that we were actu-ally, physically inside the dream, as opposed to being just a disembodied onlooker or an incomplete, surreal personality participating in the dream.
- The story or scene inside the dream would result in the imparting of something life-giving, life-affirming, or encouraging to the individual. Even if the develop-ment and progression of the dream is intense, fearful, or uncertain, its conclusion should still resonate in a life-giving way.
- **Most importantly, the essential qualities of the dream, especially its conclusion or resolution, should be consistent with Scripture or scriptural prin-ciples.** For example, a dream that appears to develop positively, even happily, but involves the subject in a direct violation of a scriptural principle (murdering, stealing, etc.), would not be sent from God.
- Any dream can be self-prompted or even implanted by the enemy. Therefore, separate confirmation(s) for the dream message should be sought or expected from other God-inspired sources. Such confirmations would be received for any legitimate spiritual dream, word, prophecy, or tongue. I had no idea how (or if)

I might receive confirmation for this dream. (What else was new?)

When I awoke from my dream, I immediately thought of two scriptural references that seemed to, thematically, describe the images in the dream.

- **Therefore since we are surrounded by such a great cloud of witnesses... (Hebrews 12:1).** This passage described how I felt under the gaze of the other businesspeople in the conference room as I engaged the CEO.
- **Mark 7:24-30, which tells the story of the Syrophoenician woman who came to Jesus to ask healing for a demon possessed daughter.** Jesus appeared to deliberately mock her, or reject her, by saying, **"First let the children eat all they want, for it is not right to take the children's bread and toss it to their dogs [the Syrophoenicians]"... But, not to be put off, the woman replied. "Yes, Lord, but even the dogs under the table eat the children's crumbs."** She had given a bold reply to Jesus' comment; a comment designed to test her. Then Jesus said, **"For such reply, you may go; the demon has left your daughter."** In the dream, I felt like the CEO was testing or questioning me (even baiting me) in a similar manner. It occurred to me that, in a sense, he was waiting for a bold answer, like the Syrophoenician woman gave Jesus, before endorsing me to his colleagues.

*(Note: When I wrote this account some 4 1/2 months later, I re-read the **Hebrews 12:1** passage, but carried on in the text just a little further. With my written memories to prompt me, and with the Spirit continually unveiling new truth, **the rest***

*of verse 1 and the beginning of verse 2 cause my heart to stir again. I now see an even more vivid image of my dream.* **"Therefore, since we are surrounded by such a great cloud of witnesses, let us throw off everything that hinders and the sin that so easily entangles, and let us run with perseverance the race marked out for us. Let us fix our eyes upon Jesus, the author and perfecter of our faith..."** *The CEO and I sure looked at each other intently as I tried to persevere under his intense questions [perhaps, the "race" he had me running]. I don't want to say that I was actually talking to Jesus in my dream. It's just fascinating and joyful to imagine that I might have been.)*

While I wondered whether or not I would receive any confirmation for this dream, I reflected upon the journey so far. It was now appearing as if my extraordinary experiences with God's *rhema* words (I was still struggling with my faith about all of this) were moving along **two distinct but parallel courses.**

- I was receiving words of encouragement and healing, **specifically for my own illness,** right down to details that had personal, experiential meaning for me ("neck," "markers," "cast idols," "shaped like a man").
- I was also receiving a broader, spiritual picture of the disease itself; a description of its overall existence. It was a picture, not just of a common physical disease, but also of an evil, spiritual stronghold. It was a stronghold (or empire) carefully constructed by the evil one to delude mankind with its institutional legitimacy. Hidden inside the earthly, healing institution was a spiritual "institution" designed to enslave, torture, kill, and process victims and families with quiet, lethal efficiency.

Inside this spiritual picture, there were also two intense **sub-issues** that increased my emotion and anticipation as I waited for more wisdom and insight.

- Just like Hope's "word" from the Lord, the recent scriptures describing the stronghold of the cancer idol had contained definite indications of the Lord's "jealousy" or anger with the idol. The scriptures also contained a corresponding promise of destruction for the idol and its stronghold. These images were separate from the promises of personal healing and restoration. It was more of a general statement of God's intention to deal with **the whole** situation. Perhaps it represented some kind of new, sweeping act of healing in "the last days." My hopes for this new move of God increased as time went on. This was especially true after I commenced treatment and experienced first-hand other cancer victims and other cancer stories. Was God finally getting "fed up" with cancer?
- The question of God's omnipotence or absolute sovereignty over everything invariably raised other questions about how this particular stronghold was "allowed" to grow so powerful and so deadly. The incredible power of cancer had caused many believers to quietly lose hope in God's ability to overcome and heal, except through a merciful and peaceful death. I guess it was still quite conceivable that this was actually God's will. No demon or evil spirit, even Satan himself, was supposed to be a match for the power of God. However, if cancer, in all its lethal power, represented God's will, then why did all the scriptural *rhema* that I was receiving contain "evidence" that He was angry? That is, if it **was** actually *rhema*.

Perhaps it was just my own wishful delusion at work. You can see my dilemma.

I was about to be "let in" on more of the secret.

# CHAPTER 16

# THE PERSONALITY OF EVIL

It was open Bible reading time again, and just a few days now until my treatment commenced. I found myself turning through the pages of **2 Kings**, until my eyes came to rest on the heading **"Hezekiah King of Judah" (2 Kings 18).** I think I originally paused here because I remembered reading about Hezekiah, some fifteen years earlier, during my journey through Chronic Fatigue Syndrome. I recalled the story of **Hezekiah's illness (2 Kings 20:1-11),** where, having been stricken with a disease, Hezekiah is informed by the prophet Isaiah that the Lord has ordained him to die. Hezekiah cried out to God for mercy, and the Lord relented, granting Hezekiah fifteen more years of life. I further remembered how this story had given me much hope during my first illness, with its picture of a God who appeared to be willing to change His mind in response to fervent prayer. Apart from this particular story, I knew nothing more about Hezekiah.

So I just scanned through the first few verses of 2 Kings 18 and picked up some background on Hezekiah:

-   **He was favored by God for conducting himself in a manner comparable to David (2 Kings 18:3).**

- He opposed the worship of idols, and destroyed the altars and symbols of idolatry (2 Kings 18:4).
- He was at war with the King of Assyria (2 Kings 18:7, 13).

These basic facts about Hezekiah drew me deeper into the scripture. The images of idolatry, combined with references to Assyria, achieved yet another connection to the story that God had been unfolding over the last few weeks. As I read on, I came to the heading, **"Sennacherib (King of Assyria) Threatens Jerusalem" (2 Kings 18:17-37).** I was not prepared for the new insights I was about to receive *(Note: This same story is related in 2 Chronicles 32:9-24 and Isaiah 36:1-22).*

The passage recounts the story of the Assyrian attack on Jerusalem. More importantly, it is a record of **the dialogue that took place among the combatants, the prophet Isaiah, and God Himself.** The passage reveals not only the bare facts of what was said and done, but provides vivid insight into **the emotions and attitudes** of all the participants (including God). As was the case with my other *rhema* experiences, reading the text seemed to illuminate the deeper, spiritual picture of cancer. To add to my amazement, the text also seemed to be giving specific answers to some of the lingering questions that had been raised in my doubting but inquisitive mind. The story begins by describing the Assyrian army amassed outside the gates of Jerusalem, ready to communicate the terms of surrender. I found myself spiritually imagining the demon of cancer threatening **my "fortified city" (Jeremiah 1:17-19),** my own body and soul. I invite the reader to "see" and imagine with me.

- **The field commander said to them, "Tell Hezekiah: This is what the great king, the king of Assyria, says: On what are you basing this confidence of**

**yours? You say you have strategy and military strength - but you speak only empty words. On whom are you depending, that you rebel against me? Look now, you are depending on Egypt, that splintered reed of a staff, which pierces a man's hand and wounds him if he leans on it!" (2 Kings 18:19-21)** I "heard" the demon responding to modern man's pronouncements about the effective treatments and "strategies" to fight cancer. These pronounce-ments often seemed like "empty words" to the victims. The image of "Egypt" as a "splintered reed of a staff" reminded me of intravenous chemotherapy. This medical "ally" also "pierces a man's hand" and "wounds him if he leans on it," through the additional burden and despair of chemotherapy side effects.

- **And if you say to me, "We are depending on the Lord our God" - isn't he the one whose high places and altars Hezekiah removed, saying to Judah and Jerusalem, "You must worship before the altar in Jerusalem?" (2 Kings 18:22)** The Bible informs us that Hezekiah was merely trying to purify the worship of the true God. He was forbidding the use of former sites of **combined** Yahweh and idol worship. Spiritually, I heard the demon reminding us that we had ourselves diluted, misused and reduced the importance (and the power) of our own God in this important battle with cancer. We have done this with the best of intentions: peaceful co-existence with the world. We had created our own "high places" of combined "worship". They were places to comfort-ably worship both the idol of science and "God-lite."

- **"Come now, make a bargain with my master, the King of Assyria" (2 Kings 18:23).** All cancer victims struggle with the idea of "bargaining" for our lives. We helplessly put this question to the cancer institution (the idol): "If I put my trust in you, can you save my life? Will you save my life?"

- **"Furthermore, have I come to attack and destroy this place without word from the Lord? <u>The Lord himself told me to march against this country and destroy it!</u>"** (2 Kings 18:25) I stopped and drew in my breath when I read this. We had gradually become convinced that the dreaded cancer process, from affliction through tortuous treatment, and finally, unto death, was **an act of God's sovereign will.** Our "spiritual" assumption was that the whole business had God's "permission." This assumption was so much easier, and faith-friendly, than the alternative option, which is to pray and believe that healing was actually God's will for us. At the end, almost all believers, victims, caregivers, and observers listen to the demon's justification that "the Lord himself told me...to destroy." Believing that it was God's will was just easier. Was this always the truth? Or, were believers often participating in their own delusion?

- **Then the commander stood and called out in Hebrew: "Hear the word of the great king, the king of Assyria!...Do not let Hezekiah deceive you...Do not let Hezekiah persuade you to trust in the Lord when he says, The Lord will surely deliver us; this city will not be given into the hand of the king of Assyria" (2 Kings 18:28-30).** The delusion is made even stronger when the demon calls out to believers in familiar, religious language and tones ("Hebrew"). This religious "calling out" is sometimes through well meaning friends and pastors who subtly urge victims to give in, to surrender to "God's will." There is often quiet pressure to cease struggling and to peacefully succumb to the "spiritual victory" to be found in God's eternal rest. (I know that this is a complicated situation. Who could argue that it is wrong to cease struggling and trust God? But, are we always surrendering to the right "god"?)

*(Note: **Then they called out in Hebrew to the people of Jerusalem who were on the wall, <u>to terrify them and make them afraid</u> in order to capture the city. They spoke about the God of Jerusalem as they did about the gods of the other peoples of the world – the work of men's hands [2 Chronicles 32:18-19]** A couple of months later, I read this alternate account of the previous text. It enhanced my understanding of how powerful the cancer delusion has become **inside** the community of believers. The scripture echoes the familiar tones of friends, family, and pastors who feel just as lost and powerless against the demon of cancer. We often mask our secret fears about the absence of God's power inside our comments about "God's will" for the cancer victim. When cancer victims hear these spoken tones, the frequent result isn't peace, but turmoil, fear ["to terrify them"] and resignation. In the process of speaking in godly, but defeated, language, we often don't realize that God's powerful healing message is relegated to the same, precarious status as surgery, radiation, chemotherapy, psychology, or alternative therapies, i.e., "the gods of other peoples...".)*

- **"Do not listen to Hezekiah. This is what the king of Assyria says: Make peace with me and come out to me. Then every one of you will eat from his own vine and fig tree and drink water from his own cistern, until I come and take you to a land like your own, a land of grain and new wine, a land of bread and vineyards, a land of olive trees and honey. <u>Choose life and not death!</u>"** (2 Kings 18:31-32) Still speaking in reassuring, "godly" tones, the demon is building the case for the victim to place complete faith in the cancer idol ("make peace and come out to me"). Why would we trust in some unrealistic, spiritual remedy (God's healing power), when you can see that mankind has built a healing system that you can touch and feel ("his own vine and fig tree and drink water from his own cistern")? The idol is your best chance for healing ("take you to a land" … "of grain … new wine…bread …vineyards …olive trees … honey). I was struck by the irony of the idol uttering the same words that God spoke in **Deuteronomy 30:19** to warn the Israelites from "bowing down to other gods" (Deuteronomy 30:17-18): **"Choose life…"** The idol even sounded like God.

- **"Do not listen to Hezekiah, for he is misleading you when he says, The Lord will deliver us. Has the god of any nation ever delivered his land from the hand of the king of Assyria? Where are the gods of Hamath and Arpad? Where are the gods of Sepharvaim, Hena, and Ivvah? Have they rescued Samaria from my hand? Who of all the gods of these countries has been able to save his land from me? How then can the Lord deliver Jerusalem from my hand?" (2 Kings 18:32b-35)**
This passage started to define the boastful arrogance of the demon. No longer content to speak in soothing, inviting tones to the victim, the demon finally shows his pride, born of a history of defeated victims ("Has the god of any nation ever delivered his land from the hand of the king of Assyria?"). As the countries were named, I pictured different human victims, all depending on different "idols" to bring them healing from cancer (conventional, alternative, or quack therapies). To varying degrees, all the "idols" participated in the process. First, by raising a victim's hope, and then, prompting despair later on. God is often viewed

as an acceptable, but mostly secondary, "positive thinking" therapy. In some ways, God is not viewed much differently from other alternative or psychological supplements to "real medicine" ("How then can the Lord deliver Jerusalem from my hand?") So, why would our appealing to yet another "god" (even the true God) result in any different outcome?

- **But the people remained silent and said nothing in reply, because the king (Hezekiah) had commanded, "Do not answer him" (2 Kings 18:36).** I wrestled with this passage for a while, finally thinking that it represented the futility of "arguing" or "defending" a position which refutes the claims of the idol. As time went on, and my treatment progressed, it became clearer that trying to explain the spiritual foundation, the spiritual battle, and the potential healing opportunity for cancer was difficult and sometimes exhausting. This was the case with cynical believers and non-believers alike. Until God identified and enabled the right timing for such an explanation, perhaps it was better not to say anything ("the people remained silent"). Or, perhaps we are not supposed to engage in a spiritual battle that God Himself wants to fight ("Do not answer him," because "I AM" will answer him?)

As I reached the end of 2 Kings 18, I was (again) reeling from the spiritual images of the cancer stronghold, which connected so well to the previous messages God had shared with me. But there were also some **new images, and new detail** which seemed to expand the understanding and increase the contemporary relevance of the images (like a modern parable).

- There was new confirmation that God, indeed, had something to do with the initial existence of the disease. I mean, it was biblically accepted that God had "raised up" rogue nations or adversaries for His people. This occurred when His people became disobedient, and especially when they turned to worshipping other gods. God's motives for raising up an enemy were, normally, chastening and discipline. The chastening was often severe, but generally it stopped short of uncontrolled destruction of His people (the Great Flood notwithstanding). Mercy and restoration were generally the ultimate intent. But, if the statement, **"The Lord himself told me (cancer) to march against this country and destroy it" (2 Kings 18:25b)** was consistent with the biblical picture of chastening and restoration, what made this cancer adversary different from others? What made this disease different from other diseases? Why had there been so few, real "cures" found? What had enabled this disease to be built into an embedded, cultural institution; a clinical and spiritual killer? **Where was the intended, post-chastening mercy and restoration?**
- The 2 Kings 18 experience produced the image of **a demon with an attitude.** It was an arrogant and proud spirit. It possessed incredible power to deceive, terrify, and overwhelm ordinary people. This demon even used God's words ("Choose life...") to convince victims to surrender to him. It was still too early to conclude anything, but this attitude suggested an extraordinary "will" to construct a spiritual and temporal machine to "kill and destroy." The sheer size and magnitude of the global cancer establishment attested to that.

I was compelled to read on into **2 Kings 19.** My mind was turning over with the new information and new insight that Chapter 18 had provided. I was not at all sure how this particular biblical account would turn out. I wondered if the story would have any direct resonance with the book of Nahum. Perhaps this wasn't the proper time in biblical history for the Nahum prophecy to be literally fulfilled. One thing I did realize, as I turned the page into Chapter 19, was that God was providing richness and depth to this spiritual picture of cancer. This new depth was directly answering some of the specific questions that had been raised by the more generalized scriptures and images received earlier in the journey. **It was as if I was being taught, step by step, by a very patient and diligent Teacher.**

**2 Kings 19 begins with the heading, "Jerusalem's Deliverance Foretold."** I was anxious to understand more about the actual events or acts of God that would accomplish this future deliverance. And, of course, I was hoping to see if the text contained further spiritual connections that might provide a deeper understanding of how a similar deliverance from cancer might be accomplished.

**2 Kings 19** focuses on the reactions and responses of Hezekiah, the prophet Isaiah, and most importantly, those of the Lord toward the threats from the King of Assyria. **To my complete amazement, the chapter explained, in vivid detail, the key underlying reasons for the rise of the cancer stronghold.** It also suggested a relationship to other historical, demonic strongholds, like the Holocaust. Just as important, the chapter began to explain how a sovereign God interacts and contends with such demonic opposition. Finally, and happily, the chapter also demonstrates how God plans to deal with such strongholds in order to carry out His ultimate plan of healing and redemption for mankind. It was so early in my journey, that, even in retrospect, it's kind of amazing that God felt that I was ready for all of these new concepts. Nevertheless, it happened, and these scriptures prompted a new, powerful flood of battle images.

- **When King Hezekiah heard this, he tore his clothes and put on sackcloth and went into the temple of the Lord (2 Kings 19:1).** I'm not sure that my own very first reaction to the news of cancer was to fall, in humility, before God. However, it's clear that all the Internet research and clinical information I gathered at the beginning, bleak as it was, eventually did "clothe me in sackcloth" and send me to the Lord. In the same way, after staring at the invincible army of Assyria for a while, Hezekiah knew what to do.
- **And they told him [Isaiah], "This is what Hezekiah says: This day is a day of distress and rebuke and disgrace, as when children come to the point of birth and there is no strength to deliver them. It may be that the Lord your God will hear all the words of the field commander, whom his master, the king of Assyria, has sent to ridicule the living God, and that he will rebuke him for the words the Lord your God has heard. Therefore pray for the remnant that still survives." (2 Kings 19:3-4)** So many cancer victims reach this stage of "distress... rebuke...disgrace" when the battle is in the balance, and when the possibility or hope of healing is still flickering faintly in their spirit. Yet the oppression, both worldly and spiritual, is so overwhelming that the "birth" of hope does not occur, because "there is no strength to deliver" or keep the hope alive. This spiritual picture of the cancer demon illustrates that the demon does not come merely to <u>attack</u> God's people which, according to the biblical text, is actually God's **initial** will. The demon also comes to "ridicule the living God;" To not just destroy

Jerusalem, but to "rub God's nose in it" and mock Him, belittling His power. **It is this arrogance that sets this enemy of cancer apart.** It is the boasting of the enemy, supported by cancer's deadly body count that not only imparts extraordinary fear to its victims, but, quite properly, draws a "rebuke" of some kind from an offended God. The phrase, "the remnant that still survives" was a new concept. It would reoccur and gain meaning as my journey continued.

- **Isaiah said to them, "Tell your master, 'This is what the Lord says: Do not be afraid of what you have heard – those words with which the underlings of the king of Assyria have blasphemed me. Listen! I am going to put such a spirit in him that when he hears a certain report, he will return to his own country, and there I will have him cut down with the sword'" (2 Kings 19:6-7).** Ok, you don't have to be afraid because God is aware and angry ("jealous") at being "blasphemed." He would respond with a "spirit" (the Holy Spirit?). He would cause the enemy to "return to his own country" (physical healing, shrinkage, remission?). He would "cut him down with the sword" (final cure through the Word of God, not just clinical medicine?).

- **Now Sennacherib [king of Assyria]…sent messengers to Hezekiah with this word: "…Do not let the god you depend on deceive you when he says, 'Jerusalem will not be handed over to the king of Assyria.' Surely you have heard what the kings of Assyria have done to all the countries, destroying them completely. And will you be delivered? Did the gods of the nations that were destroyed by my forefathers deliver them?" (2 Kings 19:9-12)** It's truly ironic when a "prince of lies" warns us not to "let the god you depend on deceive you" (God cannot lie) via the divine promise of healing and deliverance. It's not surprising that we waver in our beliefs (I know I continued to struggle) when confronted with the long, deadly history of cancer through the generations (my father, Lori's mother, so many others). This generational history was being represented by the scriptural reference to all the successive "kings of Assyria" and "all the countries ... destroyed by my forefathers." It seemed like every time God increased my hope, the enemy would up the ante and remind me of the universal and generational power of cancer.

- **Hezekiah received the letter from the messengers and read it. Then he went up to the temple of the Lord and spread it out before the Lord. And Hezekiah prayed to the Lord: "O Lord, God of Israel, enthroned between the cherubim, you alone are God over all the kingdoms of the earth. You have made heaven and earth. Give ear, O Lord, and hear; open your eyes, O Lord, and see; listen to the words Sennacherib has sent to insult the living God" (2 Kings 19:14-16).** There it was again. An image of what we are supposed to do when presented with the "idol's report" on our cancer condition. Go "up to the temple of the Lord and spread it out before the Lord." Unless we were to learn that **every** cancer death was truly "God's will," **His sovereignty** "over all the kingdoms of...heaven and earth" was being portrayed here as **the hope of victory over the enemy.** This was an enemy that spoke words "to insult the living God." Cancer's deadly dominion over us is that same "insult" to God.

- **"It is true, O Lord, that the Assyrian kings have laid waste these nations and their lands. They have thrown their gods into the fire and destroyed them, for they were not gods but only wood and**

stone, fashioned by men's hands" (2 Kings 19:17-
18). Time and time again, cancer has conquered
mankind's – self-invented, –self-fashioned "gods" of
treatment. Had I said earlier that the "monster" was
being fought with sticks and rocks? God reminded me
of this as I read the words "only wood and stone."

- "Now, O Lord our God, deliver us from his hand,
so that all kingdoms on earth may know that you
alone, O Lord, are God" (2 Kings 19:19). As we
begin to realize that our own idols of healing cannot
heal us completely, God wants us to turn to Him for the
real cure. Inside this passage, again, was an indication
of deliverance or healing beyond my own situation. It
was an indication of deliverance that "all the kingdoms
on earth may know." My heart soars at the thought of
God pouring out a global kind of healing over cancer.

The next section of 2 Kings 19, headed "Isaiah
Prophesies Sennacherib's Fall," contains God's response
to the boasts and threats of Assyria, and to the sincere prayers
of Hezekiah. For the first time in my journey, I began to
understand the relationship between God's will and the
stronghold of cancer. In "God's own words" I was being
shown the unseen subtext in the eternal battle, and how this
subtext contributed to our confusion in the temporal struggle
with cancer. We are terrorized and overwhelmed by its
unearthly power (we really don't have an earthly chance),
and, at the same time, we are accepting of the slavery it
imposes. We rationalize this struggle by thinking it MUST
be "God's will." This rationalization is partially true and
partially a delusion. God (through Isaiah) "explained" this
paradox far better than I ever could:

Then Isaiah...sent a message to Hezekiah: "This is what
the Lord, the God of Israel, says: I have heard your

prayer concerning Sennacherib, king of Assyria. <u>This is the word that the Lord has spoken against him</u>" (2 Kings 19:20-21).

- "The Virgin Daughter of Zion despises you and mocks you... Who is it you have insulted and blasphemed? Against whom have you raised your voice and lifted your eyes in pride? Against the Holy One of Israel!"(2 Kings 19:21b-22) The insults, blasphemy, pride, and arrogance of this demon are a special affront to God.
- "By your messengers you have heaped insults on the Lord" (2 Kings 19:23). Only a demonic power with an overwhelming **self-confidence** would not only insult, but "heap" those insults on God Himself. Who would do such a thing, believing they could actually get away with it?
- "And you [Assyria[ have said, With my many chariots I have ascended the heights of the mountains" (2 Kings 19:23b). In its many forms, cancer has established an unprecedented, preeminent, earthly dominion of slavery, suffering, and death.
- "I have cut down its tallest cedars, the choicest of its pines. I have reached its remotest parts, the finest of its forests. I have dug wells in foreign lands and drunk the water there" (2 Kings 19:23c-24). Cancer has enslaved and killed "the best and the brightest" of mankind, young and old, male and female. There are countless victims who were full of hope and promise for the future ("tallest ... choicest ... finest"). And the "killing fields" are worldwide ("foreign lands").
- "Have you not heard? Long ago I ordained it. In days of old I planned it; now I have brought it to pass, that you have turned fortified cities into

**piles of stone. Their people drained of power, are dismayed and put to shame" (2 Kings 19:25-26).** So the notion about "God's will" is partially true. God had ordained in days of old that this enemy would be allowed to rise up to "drain, dismay, and shame" His people. But did that also mean He ordained this transformation from purposeful chastening into malicious slaughter? Did God ordain the merciless arrogance of the killer? Did God intend that this global empire of cancer would flourish and perpetuate itself?

- **"But I know where you stay and when you come and go and how you rage against me. Because you rage against me and your insolence has reached my ears, I will put my hook in your nose and my bit in your mouth, and I will make you return by the way you came" (2 Kings 19:27-28).** God had originally permitted — even prompted — the onslaught of this disease for redemptive purposes. However, **the unique personality of this enemy** corrupted the original intent of God. No longer content to just afflict and chasten, the enemy began to "rage against" God and His purposes with pride and "insolence." God will not be mocked so He (now) has promised to control ("hook ... bit") and drive out the usurper ("return the way you came").

- **Once more a remnant of the house of Judah will take root below and bear fruit above. For out of Jerusalem will come a remnant, and out of Mount Zion a band of survivors. The zeal of the Lord Almighty will accomplish this (2 Kings 19:30-31).** God had been moved to draw a line in the sand in the face of the enemy. There would be a new "remnant," "a band of (cancer) survivors" because of the Lord's reasserted control over the demon. The "bully" was about to feel the Lord's "zeal."

- "**Therefore this is what the Lord says concerning the king of Assyria: He will not enter this city... By the way that he came he will return; he will not enter this city, declares the Lord. I will defend this city and save it**" (**2 Kings 19:32-34**). This was another confirmation of the early promise to make me a "fortified city" (**Jeremiah 1:17-19**). God was going to defend me and save me. Cancer would "not enter this city" named Fred.

- **That night the angel of the Lord went out and put to death a hundred and eighty five thousand men in the Assyrian camp. When the people got up the next morning – there were all the dead bodies! So Sennacherib king of Assyria broke camp and withdrew. He returned to Nineveh and stayed there** (**2 Kings 19:35-36**). As I read about the death of the "hundred and eighty five thousand," I could see a picture of hordes of cancer cells dying inside my body under the power of "the angel of the Lord." The two connected healing stories were again being illustrated. My own cancer would "break camp and withdraw," and then return "to Nineveh" (the stronghold) to await ultimate, total destruction (God's jealous outpouring of healing over the whole disease) as portrayed in the book of Nahum. O Lord may it be soon.

*(Note. For many years, I had been praying for my four sisters, that their relationship with God would develop in a new way. I prayed for their perception of the Lord to be real. I don't want to presume to completely understand their historical relationship with God, but I was praying for a deeper experience with Him, inside the rush of their everyday lives. We had all been brought up with the same, incomplete, fable-like picture of God. Although my more definite "Christian focus" over the*

*last number of years had enhanced this picture, the journey into the life-and-death world of cancer had exposed the shallowness of my own faith. God chose to use the occasion of my illness to affect all of my sisters, forcing them to confront the issues of life, death, prayer, and the reality of God. I am so thankful to all of them [Debbie, Leslie, Kelley, Laurie Lee] for walking beside me in love and prayer.*

*One sister in particular, Laurie Lee, was also at a place of sincere hunger for God. As His timing would have it, Laurie Lee and I began, on a regular basis, to share the incredible "communication" God had established through Scripture, dreams, people, and events. Laurie Lee's search for the things of God placed her in a unique position, both as a loving listener to her brother [listening to notions that "normal people" might have seen as desperate fantasies], and as an encourager and child-like recipient of the mysteries of God. And, mysteries indeed they were.*

*One important scriptural connection that came through Laurie Lee occurred very early in the journey. After only hearing about a couple of my experiences, Laurie Lee e-mailed me a scripture that she had discovered on a Christian website which had been particularly helpful in her own recent journey. It was an extremely important scripture, because it suggested a medium or mechanism for what was happening to me.* **"But when he, the Spirit of truth, comes, he will guide you into all truth. He will not speak on his own; he will speak only what he hears, <u>and he will tell you what is yet to come</u>" [John 16:13].** *I have to admit that I was amazed at the literal notion expressed in this passage. The Holy Spirit was actually orchestrating all of these events to communicate God's truth to me and to give me a view of the future; my future – or the future of mankind, perhaps. I was reluctant to completely embrace this notion at that moment [gee, I wonder why?], but my hopes were raised considerably to think that the Holy Spirit might be behind it all.)*

# CHAPTER 17

# THE ENEMY COUNTERATTACKS

M y first day of treatment finally arrived. There had been a month or so of preparation, prayer, intense struggle, much spiritual encouragement, and even some faint assurance. I'm not sure if I was ready, but I do know that I was both weary of, and afraid of, waiting any longer. I still fought that insidious, fearful image of the cancer growing inside me, conquering more fleshly territory with each passing day. So I guess I really was ready.

As I look back on this first day, I can now "bravely" say that God used it to build my faith and confirm His words to me. As I now write about this first day, I have no choice but to title it **"The Enemy Counterattacks."** The events of this day established the magnitude, the depth, and the sheer horror of the battlefield. The demon had observed the wonder and the hope of my preparatory experiences with God, and now, he was determined to send his own message. He wished to establish that this "killing ground" belonged to him, and that the early vision of hope was merely a more horrible death, disguised and deferred.

I arrived at the cancer clinic near the specified time, and reported to the reception desk of the chemotherapy dayroom.

I gave my name to the unit clerk and was directed to the large waiting area of the unit. The room was about half full (twenty people or so). There was a television blaring from a rack on the wall, and I immediately began to feel that same, surreal uneasiness I had experienced on my very first visit. It wasn't so much an overt, dark presence as it was an atmosphere of helplessness created by everyone's effort to make believe that the uneasiness wasn't there. It was a kind of "let's act normal and maybe it will be normal" spirit. We might have all been waiting for our number to be called at the local supermarket deli, only everyone knew where we were, really. Despite the coffee sipping, the magazine reading, and the "positive" conversational tones, it was as if I could feel the longing and fear inside the room. I sensed not just my own feelings, but a collective, silent murmuring of some kind. It was like a child's meek cry for help in a dark basement. From time to time, a nurse from the dayroom would come to the waiting area, call a name, smile, and lead the patient (and companion sometimes) into the back. I had decided to read the Nahum prophecy while inside the cancer clinic, each day of my treatment, as a kind of solitary act of spiritual warfare against the suspected demon. It was intended as a quiet declaration of faith, spoken out from within the stronghold itself. Taking my Bible out, in plain view of the other patients, took a little courage. It seemed so out of place amongst the newspapers, magazines, and "Living with Cancer" pamphlets. It might have taken some courage on my part, but it wasn't the act of a faithful, pious, or noble person. It was the act of a frightened, searching, seeker of grace. I was trying to show the demon that, even as weak as we all were, **some of us** had been shown the evil truth. And, though surrounded by the enemy, a "remnant" (me, for now) still flew a tiny flag of defiance and hope. Because it would have been too much to recite Nahum aloud, I decided to pray it, silently, into the realm where I pictured the battle being fought: around me, inside me.

I remember a Muslim lady, of middle age, coming into the waiting area that first day. She was dressed in a beautiful green silk robe and sash and I noticed a black book in her hand as she walked quietly into the room. Sitting down, she draped her sash over her head, as a kind of prayer shawl I guessed, and proceeded to read from the Koran. I'm not really sure of the areas of unity or division between Islam and Christianity, but I know that I felt her reverence and faithfulness to her God as she prayed with me in the waiting room. I remember asking the Lord for mercy and healing on her behalf, in case she was praying to a substitute deity, or even if she was praying to the same God. The same demon was attacking her as well. The same demon was attacking everyone there.

Practically an hour had passed before I noticed that patients who had arrived after me were being summoned into the treatment room ahead of me. I walked over to the receptionist and inquired. I was doubly concerned because I was scheduled for my first radiation treatment immediately following my chemotherapy session. Apologetically, she informed me that they had not received any written confirmation of my appointment, and that someone was trying to track down either the paperwork or the doctor in charge so that I could receive treatment that day. She asked for my patience. As I sat down again to wait, I wondered if I was deliberately being delayed, not by an administrative mistake, but by the spiritual enemy that dominated this place. I looked around the room, which had filled up. My eyes were overcome with the sight of so many sick and weary people; some sallow-colored, some hairless already, some wearing hats or bandanas. This overwhelming image caused me to feel even more uneasy, restless, and afraid of the unknown. I kept on reading my Bible. Finally, about an hour later, a nurse appeared in front of me, holding my file. She announced, with relief, that they had tracked down the chemo order and that she had already called the radiation unit to advise them of my delay. I thanked her and followed her into the chemotherapy dayroom. I had already been there for two hours. And it was just beginning.

Nothing really prepares you for what you see inside the cancer treatment establishment (the temple of the idol). Having made the transition from "outsider" to "insider," one immediately understands why an orientation to "Cancer U" is a course of study happily avoided by those who haven't been dragged, involuntarily, inside the classroom. It's an odd combination of concentration camp (alluding to the "holocaust" imagery) and extended care facility for beloved but failing parents. It's a place where the healthy and vital (so far) compassionately say, "Yes, we know it's an unearthly horror, but let's make it as comfortable and cheerful as possible." I mean, what else can be done?

I was led into a large, sunny room, ringed with vinyl-upholstered, reclining IV (intravenous) chairs. Most of the chairs were occupied, but a few sat vacant, waiting. "Pick one," I was told by the nurse. I walked over to a chair that was somewhat secluded from the rest of the room by the high counter of the nursing station. During this brief walk to "the chair," my eyes and my spirit took in the "movie" of mini-scenes taking place in the room, all around me:

- There was an elderly woman patient, sitting and reading a magazine, while her younger companion, a daughter I thought, read her own magazine. The daughter sipped her coffee while reading, and occasionally checked her daytimer.
- There was a middle-aged man, with a breathing tube stuck right in the middle of his throat. He was fiddling and fussing with the oxygen tank connection, as it kind of tangled with his IV line. His wife was trying to help, unsuccessfully.

- There was a really young mother wearing a bandana around her visibly bald head. There was a really young baby in a stroller beside her IV chair.
- There was another not-so-young-not-so-old man, kind of in the "prime" of his life, looking tired and worn. He was talking with the nurse as she attached the IV to his arm. I overheard him talking about how many treatments he had left until he was finished. I'll wonder forever what "finished" meant for each victim that I saw.
- There was a man who could only communicate with the nurse via pen and pad that he carried with him. I wondered if he had the same kind of cancer as I had. I wondered if I would need a pen and pad soon.
- And then, there was me.

As the nurse hooked up the bag of chemotherapy agent to the pump, and as she inserted the IV needle into my vein, I began to pray. Beginning that day, each time the needle pierced or the radiation beam penetrated, I would pray, **"Lord, guide this treatment to all the cancer cells. Direct Your healing light to those cancer cells that may get missed. Protect my healthy cells. Regenerate the good cells that die as a result of this hideous treatment."** I felt the foreign coldness of the drug entering my veins. Sitting in that sunny room, filled with quiet desperation, the full reality of my situation intruded on my prayer. I was being treated for cancer. I glanced over at the electronic pump on the IV column next to my chair. **The IV delivery rate was set at 666** (really). I couldn't shrug this image off very casually, as I sensed that the enemy had orchestrated today's delay to agitate and frighten me. It was as if he wanted me to know that he was here, just as much as God was here. The difference was that this was more the enemy's domain than God's. At least it seemed that way for now. The volume rate was never set at 666 after that day. I think it was just a subtle, opening message from Satan, especially for me.

After two hours of chemotherapy and hydration, I was detached from my IV tube and sent off to radiation therapy with a cheerful farewell from the nurse that we would "do it all over again tomorrow." I had been in the "temple" for four hours now, and I was beginning to feel it.

The radiation unit of this clinic is deep in the basement, and most of the rooms are lined in rows down various corridors of the basement. There are no windows to the outside in this area, so the corridors seem narrower, darker, and more claustrophobic than normal, despite the special "natural lighting." As I reached the waiting area of the radiation unit designated to treat me on that day, I also (simultaneously) entered a spiritual area, an "antechamber" perhaps, that had to be closer to the **"lions den" (Nahum 2:11).** As I sat down, I found myself with two female patients and their companions. The first patient was in a wheelchair, dressed in a tracksuit that couldn't hide her skeletal condition. A gray weariness seemed to cover her face, and her sad eyes just looked blankly at me, or rather, through me. Her gaze didn't strike me as envious of my (temporary) healthy appearance. She was just no longer able to look to me for sympathy or even acknowledgement. Like the wheelchair, life itself was just propping her up. Her eyes were windows into an inner lifelessness that was just waiting for her defeated body to catch up. I looked at her companion; a son, or a husband? I couldn't tell. He just added to the horror with his accepting, detached silence, a magazine covering his face. I knew he couldn't help it. What was anyone supposed to say at this stage? He was just there to "play out the hand" to the end (I saw so much of that over the next few months).

The other victim was a "youngish" woman in a grey overcoat and woolen winter hat. Her companion was an older woman; perhaps her mother or a friend. In the dim light of the waiting room, I could see that she had undergone some kind of radical, oral-facial surgery. Her mouth and jaw were severely disfigured and scarred, and she spoke in a kind of sad, lisping melody born of incredible pain and a growing burden of hopelessness. A radiation technician entered the waiting room and started speaking to this sad woman about her upcoming radiation treatment. The room was so small that the conversation could not be kept private, and if the enemy's purposes were to be considered, it wasn't meant to be private anyway. The nurse began to tell the woman that in order for her treatment to be effective, she had to continue to wear a certain type of appliance on her head during radiation (likely, her mask). The woman was protesting, begging really, if she could be allowed to continue treatment without the appliance. It had begun to irritate and chafe the already sensitive skin of the treatment area, to the point where (in her words) "the flesh was already raw and bleeding." The technician gently explained that the appliance was designed to make the woman's treatment more effective, and that they would try to alter the device to make it more comfortable, or at least bearable. The poor woman began to plead with the technician to speak to the doctor in charge, and to find a way to administer treatment without the painful appliance. The woman began to weep as she pleaded. We began to silently weep with her. Finally, the technician had to be firm. She had spoken to the doctor, and had been told that treatment could not be continued without the appliance. This was obviously not the first time it had been discussed. There was the horrible choice; wear the pain-inflicting appliance and be treated, or receive no treatment at all. The woman lowered her head in defeat. I was overwhelmed with sorrow for both the victim and technician. What was either of them supposed to do? Where was the compassion inside this problem-with-no-solution? Would the extra torture endured by this woman result in anything positive? Was there any point to the treatment at all, other than to inflict further pain and destroy hope? I pondered the incredible sorrow I felt for these women and the sense of futility that was drowning us in that room. I was reminded of Nahum, and how the Assyrians cruelly mutilated and tortured their victims before they killed them. And, I could hear the demon laughing at us. His purposes were being fulfilled inside his temple. This was his Nineveh, his house.

I was still deep in sadness when my name was finally called by the radiation technician. I followed her cheerful, energetic gait (she wore running shoes; they all did) into the radiation treatment room. This was my first time in this place. It reminded me of some kind of old science fiction movie. There was the treatment table, complete with bolts and clamps at the head. Dominating the room was the massive radiation equipment, designed to move and rotate around the body so as to direct its "healing beams" at precisely the right spot. Along the walls, radiation masks stared with empty gazes from their shelves. I was the mad scientist's experiment. As I stripped off my shirt and lay down on the cold table for the first time (another first time), I experienced another "reality check" from the enemy. I sensed that he had orchestrated all the delays and special "timing" of this first day. This was required to specifically increase my apprehension level, so that I would experience the maximum impact of that scene in the waiting room. All this "preparation" had succeeded in shifting my perception from cancer treatment to cancer "death sentence." But the best part of the demon's "special initiation day" was still to come.

The technicians (there were two every time) cheerfully and methodically shifted my body on the table, lining up the targeting laser beam of the radiation machine to the black marker line drawn on my chest. It was time for my mask to be fitted. Just before they placed it over my face, I remembered that the dentist had instructed me to wear the two molded, silicone jaw splints during each radiation session. You might remember that this would help prevent excessive radiation reflection and burning of tissues around the teeth. (You will also recall that I had to fill these splints with fluoride every night of treatment, and wear them to prevent wholesale dental destruction.) I retrieved these splints from my coat, inserted them in my mouth, and lay back down on the table. The lining up procedure was repeated. I didn't realize just how much the dental splints would change the shape of my face (like stuffing your mouth with cotton or food), until the technicians started bolting down the mask. Remember that I had agreed to participate in a clinical trial for a new, one-step, virtually opaque, plastic mask. There were small pinholes dotted throughout the surface of the mask, allegedly for seeing and breathing. I could tell that the technicians were struggling with the bolts and clamps, especially as the pressure started to increase on my face. I bravely mumbled, "I'm OK," when they asked if I was uncomfortable or not. The mouth splints had increased the size of my face. In order for the mask's preset markings to line up with the radiation beams, **the clamps had to be fastened much more tightly than in the "simulation" session without the mouth splints.** This was the demon's "coup de grace" of the day. As the final clamp was fastened, the mask felt like a heavy, leaden coffin lid that had been shut right on top of my face. The small pinholes for breathing and seeing ceased to function for either of these faculties. Abruptly, all light, and most of the air, was expelled from this tiny, terrifying space I was now in. I must have uttered some kind of whimper or noise, because I heard the technician ask me if I was all right. Once again, bravely, stupidly, I whispered through clenched teeth, "Yeah, I'll be OK for a while; except this mask is really tight." The technician tried to be encouraging and said, "I'm sorry, but it has to line up exactly with the marks, or the radiation beams won't treat the correct areas. It'll only be a few more minutes. Can you handle it for just a little longer?"

She could sense my anguish. I said, "Yes, I think so," but inside this dark, suffocating place all my loneliness, fear, and hopelessness was rising to a crescendo pitch. The technicians left the room to start the treatment, and spoke to me via the speaker system. It just made me feel more displaced, disembodied, disempowered. "OK, Fred, here we go; just a couple more minutes." I was sure I couldn't last. A few moments later, as the darkness and the suffocation overwhelmed me, I screamed silently in my mind, in my heart, but a scream nonetheless. It was a scream louder than I had ever screamed before in my life; signaling a terror that I had never experienced before. I screamed to God in the spiritual realm. I felt like an abandoned child who couldn't understand why his parents weren't there to rescue and comfort him. I felt like the final, drowning passenger on the Titanic. I was standing at the stern of a nose-diving, disappearing ship; staring into the approaching, endless depths of a cold, black ocean. I screamed for help; I cried out for grace.

Then, suddenly, mercifully, it was over. The technicians were unclamping the mask, and removing it from my sweat soaked face. Both technicians were concerned, but one of them, the female, spoke with understanding and knowledge: "We'll work on cutting some eyeholes in that mask before your next session. Maybe we can relieve some of that pressure." In my spirit, I felt as if she was saying, "I heard your scream. I've heard it before." As I put my shirt back on, I looked in the mirror at the waffle-like pattern that the mask had imprinted all over my face. These marks, deeply embedded, wouldn't fade away for the next eight hours. In my misery and fear, I thought, *How am I going to face this horror every day for the next two months? Lord, I need your help.* **I won't be able to do this on my own.** I was still in deep shock when I arrived home, and I immediately telephoned my radiation doctor's office, leaving a lengthy, thinly polite message that I wished to be withdrawn from the mask clinical trial. Since its objective was purely economic and had no direct potential medical benefits, I didn't feel the least bit guilty about withdrawing. It just wasn't worth it.

The next morning, a couple of hours prior to departure for my second day of treatment, I received a phone call from the radiation doctor's office. I was told that if I wished to withdraw from the mask trial, which was perfectly OK, I would have to be measured and fitted for another conventional, clear plastic mask. This would require another few days to schedule, and would temporarily suspend my treatment program, so I should not plan on going into the clinic that day. My chemotherapy session had already been cancelled due to these "unforeseen changes." Remembering my desperate prayer for grace the day before, my heart sank a little more. It seemed as if the enemy was still controlling the game by first putting me through the terrifying events of the preceding day, and then sabotaging my "escape route" by further delaying my already long-awaited treatment. I'm not sure if it was the Spirit of God or just some kind of inner, patient-advocacy motive to "fight the system," but I decided to go on the offensive myself. I called the radiation technicians that had worked with me the day before and told them that I would be willing to wear the experimental mask for a few more days or even longer while we waited for a new clear mask to be fitted and completed. There would be no need to completely cancel my treatment. The male member of the technical team, another compassionate, caring individual, immediately saw the logic of my idea and told me to come into the clinic right away. They could at least cut some eyeholes in the "X-mask" to relieve some of the pressure on my face. He would also call the chemotherapy department to let them know that treatment could continue. He didn't guarantee anything, but I believed his words and his tone when he promised that he would do everything possible to make it happen. With that, I headed out for my second day with the demon.

I had prayed for grace, and grace came. When I arrived at the radiation unit, the technician, with whom I had spoken earlier, came into the waiting room with a smile on his face. I wondered what other "curves in the road" would suddenly appear in this very young journey. He informed me, happily (and perhaps a little puzzled too) that they had **actually been able to find my original, clear plastic mask. For some reason, it had not been discarded,** even though the new, experimental mask had also been cast. What this meant was that I would not have to wear the dreaded "X-mask" ever again. He had arranged for a new simulation session to place target markings on the clear mask. This would take place just prior to a re-scheduled, second chemotherapy session. Chemotherapy would consume just enough time for the right settings to be calibrated on the new "old" mask. This delicate timing of events would enable me to also complete my second radiation treatment as planned. Even he seemed amazed that it had all worked out. I was more than amazed. It was difficult not to weep, out of gratitude to him, his assistant, and to my merciful God, who had clearly heard the miserable cry of his frightened child. The complicated choreography of the second day came off as smooth and dream-like as the first day had been a slow motion, living nightmare. My most acute memory of Day Two was the feeling of space and the awareness of light as they clamped the clear mask down on my face, with its large openings for my eyes and mouth. In spite of the continuing stream of new, dark images in my cancer movie, my memory of the second day is forever defined by this incredible demonstration of answered prayer and God's grace. Perhaps most importantly, this day was a statement of God's sovereignty inside the temple of the cancer idol. God had truly given me **"immeasurably more than all we ask or imagine, according to his power" (Ephesians 3:20).**

As I drove home from the clinic still pondering the incredible mercy of God, I was suddenly convicted with a new appreciation of the awesome and impossible task facing the men and women of the cancer establishment as they fight the disease, day in and day out. As scientific people, I could see how necessary it was for them to believe that all they were fighting was a monstrously deadly disease, even though I could sense that many of them suspected there was more to the story. For that reason, I knew that these same, dedicated clinicians would find it very difficult to believe that they were also contending with a powerful spiritual enemy. The notion wasn't just unscientific; it wasn't even sensible. It is this essential tension, between the spiritually aware and unaware, which has kept God officially out of the cancer healing equation. God is barely mentioned except as a helpful, psychological support mechanism, or worse, as part of the rationalization that encourages the quiet surrendering unto death. I know that I have expressed my admiration for all the caregivers of cancer, and I will again. The compassionate, skillful, even loving efforts of these unsuspecting inhabitants of "the temple" to ease my suffering would be a continued gift that I would receive from all of them throughout my long treatment. These people are a blessing to all the victims who have to enter through the gates of the temple for possible "sacrifice."

*(Note: I would recall how many times in the eyes of the caregivers, fighting cancer was like fighting a monster with crude weapons of sticks and rocks. When I got home, I re-read the passage from **2 Kings 19** that had spoken so powerfully about the arrogance and self-glorification of the demon: **"It is true, O Lord, that the Assyrian kings have laid waste these nations and their lands. They have thrown their gods into the fire and destroyed them, for they were not gods but only wood and stone, fashioned by men's hands." (2 Kings 19:17-18).** I experienced another Spirit-induced insight, connecting with Sandra Kennedy's teaching*

*about the cooperation between conventional treatment and spiritual "treatment." Conventional treatments are the "wood and stone" idols, if we depend **solely** on them for healing. Modern cancer treatments are still somewhat medieval as they torture and mutilate victims, even while healing. These "gods of wood and stone," or the sticks and rocks as I called them, are still an essential part of God's total plan for healing. I think that Dr. Kennedy's thesis, which I generally agree with, is that modern medicines and medical techniques are just another gift of healing from God. In spite of my hatred for the potential, debilitating side effects of cancer treatment, **my positive experiences with those who administered the treatment** caused me to ponder the true worth of those "sticks and rocks." Then I remembered, or rather, was prompted to remember, **the story of David and Goliath, and how David killed the giant with <u>a stone</u>, guided by the Lord.** From that moment, my attitude toward my impending treatment changed quite a bit. I came to a place where I realized that God would use whatever combination of temporal and spiritual processes to heal us. All of the processes are guided and empowered by Him.)*

## CHAPTER 18

# NOTE TO DREAMWEAVER: "AIRSICKNESS BAG PLEASE!"

A s if to punctuate the message and the power of that second day, God provided one more enormous gift to me that very evening. I received a long, voicemail message from my pastor and friend, Warren. In the message, Warren told me that he had been studying **Exodus 32, the story of Moses, the Israelites, and the golden calf.** The story had impacted Warren in a profound way, especially in the description of Moses' intercession before God for the idolatrous Israelites. Moses' fervent pleading had persuaded the Lord to relent and spare the Israelites from His wrath. Warren told me that he had been moved to intercede for me before the Lord in the same way, with the same passion and expectancy. He ended the message by encouraging me to explore the Exodus passage. As always, I was heartened by Warren's sincere care, and I opened my Bible to the **book of Exodus** and read Chapter 32. For some reason, I decided to read on into **Chapter 33** as well. I think I did this because the golden calf story seemed to draw me into the larger story about idolatry that God seemed to be sharing with me.

I reached **Exodus 33:7,** which began a section called **"The Tent of Meeting."** I grew more interested, as this section described the place and circumstances under which Moses was able to actually meet and speak with God. Beyond the story of the burning bush, I didn't realize that Moses had regular, ongoing access to God through this meeting place (The Tent), so I was quite fascinated with the ensuing story. As I read on, I reached a section, beginning at **Exodus 33:12,** entitled **"Moses and the Glory of the Lord."** Here's what I read.

**Moses said to the Lord, "You have been telling me, 'Lead these people,' but you have not let me know whom you will send with me. You have said, 'I know you by name and you have found favor with me.' If you are pleased with me, teach me your ways so I may know you and continue to find favor with you..." The Lord replied, "My Presence will go with you..." Then Moses said to him, "If your Presence does not go with us, do not send us up from here. How will anyone know that you are pleased with me and with your people unless you go with us?"...And the Lord said to Moses, "I will do the very thing you have asked, because I am pleased with you and I know you by name"** (Exodus 33:12-17).

- I sat stunned (again) for a few moments, trying to digest the spiritual picture of this encounter as it melded into my vivid memory of **the dream** about the business presentation that I had experienced a couple of weeks previous, which I remembered in detail, even though I don't usually remember dreams:
- In that dream I was in a serious conversation with an older senior executive, the CEO who was testing me.
- I was aggressively but wisely trying to win his "favor."

- All eyes were focused on him; his "presence" in the room was central.
- After the intense questioning and answering, the CEO laughed and expressed his "pleasure" with me as his associates listened intently.
- Because of his obvious approval, I knew that I had won the contract, and that everything was going to be all right.
- The CEO in the dream had looked at me and **ASKED ME WHAT MY NAME WAS**. I had told him. **He now "knew me by name."**

I remembered that the Internet site on Christian dream interpretation had specifically mentioned that a true, divinely–sent dream would somehow be **confirmed** in a Spirit-inspired, scripturally consistent manner. Now, after an inspired prompting from Warren to read Exodus, I was receiving such a confirmation from God's own words inside the Tent of Meeting. It was almost too much for me. Even as I write this account now, months later, it is still almost too much for me.

In those first days of treatment, God accomplished good things, with good timing, through these incredible demonstrations of His grace. As I look back, it now seems as if He was aware of the intense onslaught of the enemy in these initial stages of the battle, and because of this awareness, He wanted to make sure that the proper message of power and hope was sent in reply. God was replying to the demonic keepers of the idol and to me, who was so much in need. However, it only took a couple more days of chemotherapy to blur this clear display of heavenly power, and to add another discovery that attested to cancer's power to demoralize and defeat its intended victims.

If you recall, the chemotherapy agent that I was prescribed was meant to be a synergistic complement to radiation therapy. Thankfully, I was not going to lose my hair, but I was warned of "some nausea and discomfort." For this, I was given some very expensive anti-nausea drugs, as well as some practical advice to drink as much water as I could to "flush out my system" as quickly as possible. As the first days passed, the chemotherapy drug slowly accumulated in my body, and on the fourth day, I was ushered into the sickly, smothering world of the chemotherapy patient. There were no raw, open wounds or burns to show for one's trouble here. There was just a creeping countenance of pale lifelessness, and a deep, inner awareness of being extremely unwell. It is like nothing you will ever experience. I was a broken, instructional record on "coping with cancer." I found myself unprepared, again, for the sheer depth of experience that this treatment would bring. To any cancer patient with spiritual instincts even partially tuned, it's easy to see that chemotherapy penetrates very close to the core of one's being. It pierces deep to that inner place where the real life and death decisions are made. Your conscious mind is aware (or fighting to remain aware) that this stuff saturating your body is clinically designed to be life giving. However, your spirit is also aware, and is fighting the lingering suspicion, that this stuff is actually poison. Oh, the doctors will tell you that they, too, are aware of the severe physical and emotional price that chemo patients (and radiation or surgery patients, too) must pay through the side effects of treatment. And, there is considerable sympathy expressed by the entire cancer establishment over the (necessary) suffering that patients must endure. But, there is also a kind of weird indifference or detachment inherent in the treatment experience. It is a detachment masquerading as a wholly pragmatic question. (Remember the desperate, weeping lady in the radiation waiting room?). **Practically speaking, would you rather endure this hideous treatment, which may "possibly" save your life, or would you rather forgo treatment and die for sure?** It's your choice.

The subtle, innate cruelty of this choice under girds the spiritual foundation of the whole process. When trying to understand chemotherapy, the word "toxic," as it is used reluctantly by the medical establishment, is unfortunately and horribly accurate when spoken in conjunction with a cancer patient's spirit. The inner truth of chemotherapy is that it can sap your ability to resist the gradual, spiritual capitulation to the demon, and perhaps to death. On the eighth day from the commencement of chemotherapy, I wrote the following comment in my notes:

**"I can see another reason why the enemy is so successful at making victims give over (to death) – Chemo is poison, torture to the body, mind, spirit – Even my "mild" dose creates a kind of unwellness/despair world – Where I could see severe patients longing for relief (death) – Is relief from torture, God's mercy? (Yes...) But is the torture unto death His will, or Satan's insolence and cruelty? A process by which we have been blinded into thinking that death (relief) is God's only will. As I looked around the chemo waiting room and day room – I could only think of how far Satan has been allowed to go, with our help, to convince us that all this suffering must be God's will...it's not."**

It took me a long time to decide about the last two words in my note: **"it's not..."** I had nothing concrete, really, on which to base this rather categorical statement about God's will. I had received so much incredible information from God's Word about the spiritual basis of this disease. There had been incredible clues to the demonic activity, the spiritual stronghold and temporal institution, and even God's jealous opposition to the idol. **But, to presume to know God's will** presented a whole new challenge for one whose spiritual self-esteem was as low as mine was.

It's a debate with a "slippery slope" when you discuss the relationship between suffering, death, and God's will. There are many, diverse schools of thought on this subject, and they all seem to have a strong position. There is the camp that believes that "God will victoriously heal everyone, because sickness is a cursed lie from the enemy." At the other extreme end of the spectrum, there is the camp that believes that "God allows thorns (a la Paul's incurable "thorn"), like redemptive suffering or dying, to make us more like Christ." As for me, I feared that I was mostly basing the declaration, "It's not (God's will)" upon my own, too human brokenness over my personal situation. It also could be merely a result of the deep sympathy I felt for the many victims that I had seen so far. On the other hand, I sensed that the issue just couldn't be as coldly and statistically "cut and dried" as we were all being led to believe. In addition, there was this tenuous, still fragile stream of scriptural images and messages I had been receiving. I was pretty sure that my experiences wouldn't hold up very well if confronted with learned scriptural arguments from any of the established theological "camps." Yet, there was a deep conviction in my heart that there was still something very wrong. It was buried deep inside this gradual, attritional wearing down of the body, mind, and spirit that I was witnessing and experiencing.

*(Note: Just this one additional postscript to the chemotherapy experience. I also realized that, even at the peak of the most severe side effects, God was granting me a special grace; and it wasn't just the fact that I was going to keep my hair. I was sick enough to understand what people were going through, but not sick enough to actually want to give up. Through the discovery and reflection upon this new knowledge, God was giving me another reason to look to Him for grace and not give over to all the "voices" urging me to surrender to my fate.* **This pattern of fear and experience, balanced by vision and grace** *[I call to mind my description of the first*

*two days of treatment]* **was to define my overall journey through cancer treatment.** *Whether this balance was just God's grace or His plan for my chastening and education, or if it was because of the intercession of others, or possibly a combination of all of the above, I don't know. But, it was a pattern that was to follow me throughout my treatment.)*

I couldn't resist. Perhaps it was because I was so sick and depressed from the chemotherapy. I needed to look more intentionally for confirmation of God's involvement inside this present reality of disability and helplessness. It was very difficult to sustain any kind of extensive "open reading" or deep concentration on the Bible during this period of days. The nausea and general feelings of being unwell were at their height. So, I "cheated" a little and reached for my Cruden's Concordance. I was still a little incredulous at the dramatic connection that had been made between my "business meeting" dream and **Exodus 33:12-17 ("because...I know you by name")**. I decided to check for more confirmation that God actually dealt with people in this way. When I think about it now, what more credibility did I really need after such a miraculous connection in the first place? But, then was not now, and my need then was real. Using the key words "ask your/my name" or "know your/my name," I was led to **Genesis 32:23-30, the story of Jacob's wrestling match with God.**

- **So Jacob was left alone, and a man wrestled with him till daybreak. When the man saw that he could not overpower him...Then the man said, "Let me go..." (Genesis 32:24-26a).** In my dream I had "wrestled" verbally with the CEO; he learned he could not "overpower" me. He good-naturedly gave up (or asked to be "let go") by acknowledging my abilities and confidence.

- **But Jacob replied, "I will not let you go unless you bless me" (Genesis 32:26b).** I was tenacious and intense in my dialogue with the CEO. I wanted the "blessing" of a successful contract award.
- **The man asked him, "What is your name?" "Jacob," he answered (Genesis 32:27).** This was almost verbatim with what was spoken in my dream. In answer to the question, I remember answering the CEO the same way, by simply stating my name.
- **"It is because I saw God face to face, and yet my life was spared" (Genesis 32:30b).** I didn't want to be so presumptuous to think that I had actually seen God face to face, but it filled me with joy to think that I might have. It challenged me to believe that my life was to be spared as well.

In spite of the potential "contrivance" argument (because I used a Concordance) that might be posted later, God seemed to know my special need at that time. He was faithful to provide another confirmation of the timeless way He can deal with man. I was encouraged a little, yet again.

# CHAPTER 19

# GLIMPSES OF ANOTHER WORLD

By Day Ten, post-chemo, I was feeling well enough to function "normally" again; normally meaning not having to sit stationary for hours with my eyes closed, only rising if necessary. It also meant travelling more comfortably each weekday to the cancer clinic for my regular walking tour of the temple, and oh yeah, my radiation treatment. I had been scheduled for thirty-five radiation sessions, the maximum allowable for this particular region of my body. I was beginning to experience some of the side effects from radiation that I had been warned about a month earlier. It seemed like a long time already. My throat was not yet "more than a tonsillectomy"-sore, but I was beginning to feel the irritation. The most remarkable development was the subtle mutation of my taste buds. They told me to expect some "taste changes," but like so much of the "cancer-speak" that goes on around diagnosis, prognosis, symptoms, and side effects, the term was typically vague. "It affects people to varying degrees" was usually the best description you could get regarding side effects, unless, of course, you were looking for some encouragement. Then, a much more firm "Oh no, it will definitely get worse," or "You'll definitely need that painkiller," or, "We can also give you something stronger" kept everyone comfortably on the reality track. Perhaps the term "varying degrees" was encouragement.

The "taste changes" began, curiously, as just that: changes. The most accurate way to describe this first phase is to use the example that I employed most often during this time when I was asked about it. Imagine a typical, fast food, grilled hamburger, seasoned with some kind of salt-based meat spice. But also imagine the grill cook mistakenly picking up the wrong bottle, and instead of meat spice, he seasons the burger with nutmeg or cinnamon instead. Almost every food I was familiar with began to take on this bizarre, unpredictable flavor profile. Everything tasted different but not yet completely offensive. That unfortunate evolution would take place just a couple of weeks later. But I don't want to jump ahead too much, as I need to relate to you details of the last "lunch meeting" I would attend for the next four months or so.

You will remember that my friend Hope had been in touch with a gentleman who had been healed of a brain tumor. She had been trying to arrange a mutually agreeable time when we could all meet each other. Finally, we were able to set up a lunch meeting with this man, Jim. I wasn't sure what I was anticipating. Perhaps I was expecting some kind of first-person blueprint for seeking and receiving a healing from the Lord. After all, being healed of a brain tumor was major league stuff. It seemed almost biblical,epic, in the magnitude of the problem, I thought. A brain tumor was, arguably, even more serious than my own illness. I **was** sure that I was curious.

Lori, Hope, Don, and I met Jim at one of the local restaurants. He was a young looking man in his 40s: healthy, tanned, and confident. He reminded me of a Christian male model, smiling warmly in those photographs of happy couples or families that you see in Christian magazines and media. This is not meant as a disparaging comment, because in a way, I envied him right from the moment I saw him. I also became even more aware of the distinctions between us as he told his story to us, which was incredible in its own way. His sincerity and his seeming ease with the intense, emotional details of his journey were both disarming and disturbing to me. Perhaps it was because the details were so remote yet so intimately connected to me. It actually took him a while to even get around to telling about the brain tumor. He navigated his way through a two-year odyssey that was scarred by memories of a sister who had died of a similar brain tumor. During this same period, a personal medical crisis had strongly suggested a possible diagnosis of ALS (Lou Gehrig's Disease). Only a trip to the Mayo Clinic had confirmed that this was not the case. Then there was a series of horrible family tragedies. First, the accidental death of his nephew, and then, incredibly, the death of his brother (the father of the nephew). And finally, in the midst of all this, he received his own brain tumor diagnosis. We sat and listened as he calmly, even warmly, shared these background details to his healing testimony. I remember feeling kind of numb, then hypersensitive, and then uncomfortable with the definite and sure faith statements that he shared; these made me feel totally out of my element. Recounted here are the "pearls of great price" that he had gathered from these experiences:

- Nothing, absolutely nothing, was as important to him as was his newfound relationship with God. It was a relationship forged on the anvil of total helplessness and intense prayer.
- His total helplessness was only overcome by **his total surrender to God's will**, whatever that may be, even if it meant his own death.
- Regardless of the short-term, fleeting pleasures of earthly life, or the responsibilities and success which

such a life brings with it, he was actively, daily, **looking forward to his eternal life** and reward in heaven.

I know that I called myself a Christian, but I was truly humbled — even intimidated — as these incredible concepts came forth in his quiet story. I knew that I was definitely not this kind of Christian, notwithstanding my core belief in Jesus' saving sacrifice. If these concepts characterized or defined true Christian motivation, I had a long way to go. If the concepts were definitive preconditions to healing, I definitely had a long way to go.

Then, Jim finally talked to us about the brain tumor; it was almost an anticlimax after all he had just shared. Just a few months prior, Jim had been experiencing symptoms which resulted in a series of tests, scans, and an examination by a prominent neurologist in the city. The diagnosis had been returned; the cancer was in an early stage, but he had a potentially serious brain tumor. (You will remember that his sister had died of a similar brain tumor.) Jim told us that, despite the diagnosis, his previous trials had given him a tremendous amount of peace about the looming challenge as well as the potentially grim prospects. After the initial diagnosis, he decided that his approach was going to be guided by a complete surrender to God's will for his life. Because of the close relationship God had established with him during his past challenges, Jim was not really afraid; he had absolute confidence of his eternal safety in God. **In fact, he did not even pray specifically for healing.** That's right; he didn't even ask God to heal him.

Approximately four weeks after his initial diagnosis, Jim sat in the office of the neurologist, along with another physician, and was told that the latest scans of his brain showed that the tumor had mysteriously disappeared. Oh, did I mention that he hadn't even asked for healing? The expected drama and "fireworks" of this divine healing story never happened for me. The tumor had simply disappeared, quietly and graciously — miraculously. Jim almost apologized that there wasn't more to the healing testimony. I was too confused, puzzled, and even frustrated to do more than just politely mumble my thanks for the validation that God indeed healed cancer. The rest of Jim's story was, quite frankly, lost on me. I had to pray, reflect, and struggle with it in my own way.

**That afternoon, I pondered the rush of feelings and impressions from the lunch with Jim.**

- He hadn't asked for healing.
- He hadn't relentlessly pursued a healing knowledge of God.
- He had surrendered completely to God's will. That was like "surrendering to one's fate," wasn't it?
- He didn't exactly say that he wanted to die, but he did say "that he was looking forward to his eternal home." (He felt this way even right now as he lived in divine health.)

None of these thoughts were particularly uplifting for me; in fact, they were even a little demoralizing. Jim seemed so passive, so indifferent to living or dying. Even though I envied his courage and sense of assurance in God, I knew that, at least at this point in my own journey, I definitely wanted to live -... definitely. (I had no idea just how significantly different and how deeply authentic Jim's experience would appear just a few months later.) I was frustrated, irritated, and afraid. I feared that, by pursuing, reaching for, praying for, or crying out for healing, I might not be following the right path, the path that God "really" wanted me to follow. Perhaps I was just acting out of my own selfish, very human survival instinct, and in reality, was just setting myself up for disappointment. I mean, how could I ever expect to face my future, even my death, with the same quiet, assured faith in God that Jim had acquired (somehow)? This faith for God's sovereign hand in "any outcome" had evidently been significant in Jim's healing. I was really struggling with this until God prompted an insight from the very scriptures that I had been reading about Jesus' healing ministry (an unexpected benefit to my ongoing reading of these accounts). That evening, I wrote about this insight in my notes:

**"God brought to mind the image of Jesus' healing activity with huge crowds of needy, afflicted people – People with different approaches to seeking for healing (passive, active, vocal, visual…from different accounts of Jesus' healing circumstances) – Some, perhaps, weren't even really seeking – <u>They, perhaps, were far in the back of the crowd, not even realizing that Jesus had passed by them</u> – <u>His power healed them anyway</u> – Jim and I are just different individuals in the crowd – His experience doesn't invalidate the guidance, assurance, and the Words I have been receiving in my active search for God's healing will…I am being obedient by praying and pursuing God for healing – It's just a question of "who are you in the crowd?"**

Jim's healing testimony was a future blessing that I was yet to understand. This insight from the Spirit kept me from being frightened away from the personal, healing journey that God had chosen for me. Another interesting connection came from my recollections of Sandra Kennedy's teaching on the personal *rhema* manifestations of Jesus' healing will. She used the **examples of Jesus' various methods of healing blindness:**

- **by the victim's faith (Matthew 9:27-30)**
- **by spitting on the eyes and laying on His hands (Mark 8:22-26)**
- **by making mud with spit, and washing in a pool (John 9:1-7)**

Dr. Kennedy used these examples to illustrate the *rhema* healing event for each individual as a personalized demonstration of Jesus' (God's) general healing will. So, even though Jim had not asked for healing, I reasoned by these insights that God knew and understood (and even approved) my own current state of faith. **God was fully aware that even though Jim had not asked for healing, I would be asking.** Still, this experience would linger in my mind and spirit, continually raising questions, doubts, and often prompting other insights. I have come to believe that God timed our meeting with Jim to be an ongoing example of faith matured through trial. The memory of this meeting would continue to be an "irritant" to my hard-shelled doubts, questions, and pre-dispositions about the real truth of God. It was like spiritual "sand inside my oyster." I was aching to produce (or find) my own pearl of great price.

I spent the week after this meeting engaged in the new reality of my cancer treatment; my new life inside the stronghold. I had been going to the clinic on a daily basis for more than two weeks now, and as the days wore on and the side effects of the treatment progressed, my vision of the whole cancer "universe" progressed as well. I'm not sure if I mentioned this earlier in the notes; I'm pretty sure that I haven't. I'm curious how the individual perception of this "universe" differs by victim. I mean, there are some cancer patients who by desire, or necessity, continue to function in a completely regular, normal manner, even as they "battle" cancer; even unto death. They continue to work at their jobs, still engage in their relational or social duties with sincerity and vigor. They do their level best to make the "universe" a "normal" place for themselves, their co-workers, and their loved ones. I've heard from some victims who have chosen this path that they do so to create an aura of normalcy, which everyone seems to want. However, I suspect that an underlying motivation may have something to do with the constant and eventually exhausting fight to deny the monster its appetite for devouring "bits," and finally "chunks," of their lives.

It is a subtle but distinct difference in perception, this idea of normalcy. For an outsider, it has to do with keeping or maintaining an air that things are going to be OK. For an insider, it is about making a stand until forced to give ground, knowing that one's inability to deny the enemy its advance puts one closer, inch by inch, to the reality that things will not be OK. Without really being able to check this out empirically, I wonder if all cancer victims feel as uniquely alone as I did. It's not that I didn't have a loving and concerned family or devout and prayerful friends (even as I had limited these to a closely held few). And, it wasn't because I had chosen to cloister myself completely, because I hadn't, really. I still routinely engaged my close family members and prayer partners. I still did the grocery shopping, my banking, and the other sundry duties that required doing. Staring at all the food products lined up in the shelves and coolers at the supermarket, while I was completely unable to eat any regular food at all, remains (to this day) one of the singularly weird experiences of the journey. Even more weird was watching all of the hungry, food-enabled shoppers "hunting and gathering" their prey at said supermarket, knowing that I used to be one of them. No, the aloneness was more spiritual again than merely being separate from other people. It had more to do with our "altered status". We were no longer citizens of the "State of normal health, illness, and recovery," but rather, we were more like prisoners, secretly incarcerated for political crimes, or on some "death row" waiting list. We had been sentenced for an indefinite period of time, with an indeterminate future, subject only to the mercy of the state. It's not that you are unaware of what's going on in the normal world. You are even quite aware that you're still able to function (sort of) in the normal world. But, you are also aware that you are experiencing something in your deepest self that will forever separate you from the normal world. I know that I have said that my cancer diagnosis was God's (last resort) method of separating me from some of the spiritual garbage in my life — garbage that threatened to destroy my eternal safety. He also (reluctantly) used cancer to discipline me and teach me some important truths about my temporal life and relationships. I wasn't sure if I was a good student or not.

As I started to journey through the "heart" of my cancer treatment, I realized another consequence of this deep alone-ness. It was the phenomenon of walking inside, or beside, the Spirit of God while still completely inside the brutal reality of cancer. Being "alone with cancer" is like being transported around in some kind of transparent bubble that allows you to see and sometimes experience what normal life used to be about, but at the same time, the bubble can stifle and suffo-cate like a plastic bag over your face. Most of the time, the bubble only has enough room for your own reality and God's presence. In this way, the separateness is bearable, not as terrifying, and is even sweet at times. The bubble shrinks and suffocation sets in, when you can no longer sense that God is beside you. The suffocation gets worse when you start to believe (as so many do) that God is actually absent, or even worse, powerless to help you. As I write about this feeling now, I can see that another evil function of the cancer demon is to create this sense of complete aloneness, this void, in and around its victims. If the "bubble space" can be successfully and exclusively occupied by the stark, earthly reality of the disease (the idol), then suffocation and ultimate execution of the victim, is much easier. But the aloneness can also be used by God to focus the victim's heart squarely and singularly on Him. It's completely biblical that God uses adversity to get our attention and to convince us of our dependency on His power and grace. It's sad to admit that this (necessary) principle works; the greater the adversity, the greater the focus on God. I don't know how many times I wished that I had been a more teachable, more obedient pupil. If it had not been for God being with me, inside my aloneness, I don't know how I would have survived even the first diagnosis, let alone the next months of treatment and uncertainty. I don't wonder anymore about the hundreds of thousands of cancer victims who must face the monster alone, with only the idol (the "reality") occupying their personal void. God is calling them to healing as well. The only thing is, once you're inside the bubble, it can be even more difficult to hear His call.

On each day of treatment, I would make the twenty minute drive to the cancer clinic, park my car, and walk the rest of the way into the back entrance, which was conveniently close to my radiation unit. I would sometimes start praying as I drove up the final hundred yards to the building, wondering which cars passing by me contained cancer patients. I would sometimes start praying as I crossed the street in front of the clinic. I wondered if the people, in the cars passing by, knew or cared what was going on inside the innocent-looking building on the hill. I would often start praying as I entered the clinic and moved to take a seat in the waiting room. These acts of waiting, seeing, and praying, and not the radiation treatments themselves, became the featured events of my time at the clinic. It seemed as if, each day, God would allow me another example, insight, conviction, or shock, to reinforce the enormity of the experience I was having. At the same time, the enemy was trying to use some of these same events to demoralize and discourage me. The quiet, exquisite delusion of the cancer clinic acts as a kind of tranquilizer to the spirit of man, even as that spirit wants to cry out in need. We fight this sedation, even as the Spirit of God seeks to lift from us the growing, inner burden of weariness imposed on us by the evil spirit of cancer. There is a deliberate and contrived calm inside the clinic. This calm is echoed in the muted, coordinated colors of the walls and floors, the cheery and encouraging staff, the diligent and courteous volunteers offering you coffee or tea (if you can drink it). This "atmosphere" swirls around you as you wait for your turn and as you watch the other quiet drama of illness and suffering unfold around you. Only the ill and the suffering know how acute our mutual focus is on one another. It's a struggle to reconcile how much you begin to care (in a very selfish way, sometimes) about this unlikely, dark community, and yet feel such complete helplessness at the same time. And so, you pray.

- I remember the man whose face was so swollen by steroids, or radiation, or both, that he looked like one of those half-size, facially exaggerated puppets of famous politicians that you see on television.
- I remember seeing a married couple where the wife was on a movable bed, so weakened and tortured by treatment that she was constantly changing positions to try and relieve her discomfort. Her husband stood beside the bed, so loving, so devoted, so helpless. All he could do was hold her hand and look down at her as she lay there. He was whispering quietly to her.
- I remember the little girl, younger than my own children, with a bandana covering her head, acting just like any little girl. Her mother, worried and worn, speaking "optimistically" to a friend.
- I remember all the mothers, fathers, sons, daughters, husbands, wives …the breathing tubes inserted in

throat holes … the wheelchairs occupied by people too weak to walk, young and old …the teenage girls, dressed in the latest fashion-magazine styles, waiting for their radiation treatment …the scarred, stitched incisions on partially shaved heads …silent, discreet glimpses of the fear tucked underneath the calm.

If we could be unashamedly honest, we patients would admit to our feelings of separation from the normal world and our aloneness from others. We would also admit to being members of some kind of "family of strangers" as we watched, cared, and sometimes prayed for each other. I wonder if a group was organized to practice a form of silent, "guerilla" praying inside the cancer clinic, would the Spirit of God supplant the spirit of cancer more easily? Would we see some incredible, unexplainable, miraculous things as a result? I wonder.

You may remember that I had committed to reading the entire book of Nahum, inside the clinic, each day of my treatment. And, each day, I encountered more reasons, and more people, for which to read this "prophecy" for the destruction of cancer. I don't know if it was just because all my emotions and sensitivities were highly tuned while in there, but I often sensed the presence of God around us as we waited together for treatment and hoped together for healing.

# CHAPTER 20

# REBEL WITH A CAUSE

It was around the time of my second week of treatment that God decided to extend more of His mercy to me. In the midst of my confusion and struggle with Jim's healing story, God took advantage of my perplexed, inquiring spirit by uncovering another layer in my understanding of the cancer stronghold. A few weeks earlier, my spiritual connections with the passages in **2 Kings 18 and 19** had illuminated the first insights about the character and personality of the cancer demon, especially those traits of arrogance, pride, and insolence before God. In spite of God's original allowance for the existence of the disease, and His affirmation of its power to afflict and chasten, **the 2 Kings text clearly demonstrated that God ultimately would have to respond punitively to His own creation. "I will put my hook in your nose and my bit in your mouth, and I will make you return by the way you came" (2 Kings 19:27-28).** Now, as then, I don't want to claim to understand the significance of this rogue element in the light of God's absolute sovereignty and control over creation. But, it was clear that this spiritual rebel did exist then, just as it was being demonstrated to exist now, in the form of the cancer stronghold. In this particular chapter of the journey, I would receive confirmation of this act of **"the servant turning on the master;"** actually, it would be more than **just** confirmation. I would be given a deeper, more colorful picture of the intensity and emotion of the conflict as well. And, I would receive a fresh grip on the hope that was becoming a recurrent theme of the journey. It was a hope that was becoming a growing lifeline to me.

It was open bible reading time again, and the pages turned to the heading in **Isaiah 10:5, "God's Judgement on Assyria."** There was no doubt in my mind I had to read this. The Spirit of God started telling the story right away.

- **Woe to the Assyrian, the rod of my anger, in whose hand is the club of my wrath! (Isaiah 10:5)** There was no doubt now. God had "raised up" or allowed cancer, like any other sickness or adversity, to be His instrument of discipline.
- **I send him against a godless nation, I dispatch him against a people who anger me, to seize loot and snatch plunder, and to trample them down like mud in the streets (Isaiah 10:6).** I sensed that "godless" could mean idolatrous, as well as atheistic or disobedient. God had intended cancer to "seize," "snatch," and "trample." These were all words of punishment, humiliation, or discipline — or teaching, perhaps? But, they did not appear to be words of inescapable annihilation.
- **But this is not what he [Assyria] intends, this is not what he has in mind; his purpose is to destroy, to put <u>an end</u> to many nations (Isaiah 10:7).** So, the demon has a mind of its own and a self-willed purpose: "to destroy, to put an end to many nations (many victims)." And he was succeeding, generation after generation: Assyria, The Holocaust, cancer. An eternal destroyer.

- As my [Assyria] hand seized the kingdoms of idols, kingdoms whose images excelled those of Jerusalem and Samaria – shall I not deal with Jerusalem and her images as I dealt with Samaria and her idols? (Isaiah 10:10-11) "Godless" did mean idolatrous. The cancer enemy had been raised to discipline the idolatrous. But, wholesale death instead of discipline occurred. Was this because of the enemy's own rebellious intent, **and** the failure of the nations (people) to turn from idolatry as well? I remembered Isaiah 44: **Half of the wood he burns in the fire; over it he prepares his meal, he roasts his meat and eats his fill. He also warms himself and says, "Ah! I am warm; I see the fire." From the rest he makes a god, his idol; he bows down to it and worships. He prays to it and says, "Save me; you are my god." (Isaiah 44:16-17)**
- **When the Lord has finished all his work against Mount Zion and Jerusalem, he will say, "I will punish the King of Assyria for the willful pride of his heart and the haughty look in his eyes" (Isaiah 10:12).** Discipline and teaching was still God's intent for us. But when this "work was finished," God was going to punish the demon for his "willful pride" and "haughty look." But when?
- **For he [Assyria] says: "By the strength of my hand I have done this, and by my wisdom, because I have understanding ... like a mighty one I subdued their kings" (Isaiah 10:13).** The demon was not only boasting about his superior power, as before, but *now* he was boasting about superior "wisdom ... understanding." He possessed greater self-sufficiency and abilities "like a mighty one." (Like a god?)
- **"As one reaches into a nest, so my hand reached for the wealth of the nations; as men gather**

abandoned eggs, so I gathered all the countries; not one flapped a wing, or opened its mouth to chirp" (Isaiah 10:14).** The parallels between the histories of the Holocaust and the cancer stronghold were vivid. Often the most promising or accomplished people ("the wealth of the nations") become victims. The victims are "abandoned," and the abandonment (delusion) is worldwide ("all the countries"). The delusion is so strong, the fear so oppressive, that real spiritual resistance ("flapped a wing") is crushed. True spiritual knowledge, even dissident voices ("opened its mouth to chirp") which might actually defeat the monster, are smothered. During the Holocaust, the Jews had not run ("flapped a wing"), raised a dissenting voice ("opened its mouth to chirp), or in any way resisted the "hand" of the Nazi evil. Interesting.

- **Does the ax raise itself above him who swings it, or the saw boast against him who uses it? As if a rod were to wield him who lifts it up, or a club brandish him who is not wood! (Isaiah 10:15)** God was acknowledging that the cancer demon had turned on Him, and now sought to "raise itself above him," "boast against him," and "wield him" (control Him?). God was also confirming that the demon (and the stronghold) were built and maintained upon a foundation of idolatry (a "wooden club"). This stronghold could not presume to control ("brandish") the only One who is not a false idol, "who is not wood" — the One true God.

*(Note: I want to stop and mention here that these newest spiritual images were starting to prompt thoughts about an even deeper enemy involvement. These were not just your "garden-variety" evil spirits, like **the one that cried out at Jesus' approach [Mark 1:23-24], or like those who were***

*easily and gratefully driven into a herd of drowning pigs
[Luke 8:26-32]. I was beginning to imagine a unique kind of
demonic involvement; a force that was possessed of purpose,
pride, understanding, power, self-grandeur; a force that was
even claiming "equality" with God. I remember making a
special, mental note about the thoughts contained in Isaiah
10, and later on these thoughts would be confirmed in a
profound way.)*

- **Therefore, the Lord, the Lord Almighty, will send
  a wasting disease upon his sturdy warriors; under
  his pomp a fire will be kindled like a blazing
  flame. The Light of Israel will become a fire, their
  Holy One a flame; in a single day it will burn and
  consume his thorns and his briers. The splendor
  of his forests and fertile fields it will completely
  destroy, as when a sick man wastes away. And the
  remaining trees of his forests will be so few that a
  child could write them down (Isaiah 10:16-19).** I
  read this section, savoring the thought of God sending
  a "wasting disease" upon my own wasting disease;
  turnabout being more than fair play. I was drawn to
  the phrase "in a single day," but I was too much a
  prisoner of my circumstances (and the still prominent
  lumps on my neck) to think that the "single day" was
  any day soon. I was encouraged by the overall resonance with Nahum concerning the prophetic destruction of the cancer stronghold. I also continued to be
  encouraged by the personal way it was being given
  to me. I would find out two months later just how
  prophetic and personal these words were.
- **In that day the remnant of Israel, the survivors of
  the house of Jacob, will no longer rely on him who
  struck them down but will truly rely on the Lord,
  the Holy One of Israel (Isaiah 10:20).** Those words

"remnant" and "survivor" reconnected me with earlier scriptures (2 Kings 19). The words also gave me a sense of purpose and identity (perhaps future identity) beyond just being sick. I reflected on the images of the remnant; the survivors would not surrender to the idol of cancer. These survivors would not "rely" on the half-empty promises of the idol "who struck them down" in the first place. This reference identified the lethal nature of cancer as intertwined with the temporal establishment that unwittingly nurtures the invincible image of the disease. The survivors would survive by "truly" relying on the Lord.

- **The Lord Almighty will lash them with a whip, as when he struck down Midian at the rock of Oreb ... In that day their burden will be lifted from your shoulders, their yoke from your neck; the yoke will be broken (Isaiah 10:26-27).** What wonder I felt when God reconnected me to the story of Gideon (Midian was my first picture of cancer). What hope I felt as He personalized the healing vision for me, focusing on the lumps (the "yoke") on my neck. It was a yoke that would not only be "lifted," but would also be "broken."

# CHAPTER 21

# UNDERSTANDING

I have mentioned, numerous times in this account, how I seemed to be fighting a running "battle of thoughts" with the enemy. The demon sent, suggested, whispered, stabbed, and even shrieked thoughts of resignation and death. And, I would counter with a continual resistance and a refusal to accept these thoughts or visions of death. I continue to fight this battle of the mind today; it has not dissipated. This battle for the mind of the victim is exhausting, especially when combined with the overwhelming torrent of temporal, medical information pointing to the invincibility of cancer. Often the victim is overmatched when he tries to maintain his mental "defenses." Even when God is an important part of this mental conflict, especially in the area of faith for healing, the "balance of power" can still be very precarious. Reassuring thoughts about God's desire to heal can prevent the victim from being completely overwhelmed by the enemy's onslaught. Yet, the result is often a frustrating, uncertain debate about the nature of truth; the truth of God's Word vs. the truth of the world and the idol. This was the case for me.

I had been the recipient of numerous spiritual experiences, in real time, that pointed to an incredible truth about God's reality and power. The opposing side in the debate always sought to dilute and diminish the experiences as merely coincidence, or worse, desperate self-delusion. It seemed that, just as I was about to (mentally) apprehend my experiences as representations of truth, I would always hear those opposing "voices." They would point me to the "reality" of cancer: the statistics, the power, the wholly human experience. My own sense of unworthiness and skepticism over why God would choose to "communicate" with **me** in such a powerful way always seemed to prevent me from really staking everything on **His truth.** At the same time, I realized that my faith for this process needed to increase, if I were to have any chance of **doing my part in this healing connection with God.** I've always had a strong mind, but it seemed that, in this battle of thoughts, the best I could do was to reach a type of mental **stalemate** with the demon. I needed help, and whether I asked openly or secretly, God must have heard me. He provided another amazing connection to His reality through our friends Hope and Don, and, of course, His Word.

We had continued to gather with Hope and Don each Thursday evening to share the journey and to pray together. I looked forward to these times when I could share my experiences in a sympathetic but non-patronizing environment. I felt free to express my wonder, as well as my doubts, surrounding these incredible spiritual "coincidences." I think that everyone was contending somewhat with the credibility question, but they remained patient and attentive since I was the one who it was actually happening to and I was the only one with cancer. I remember explaining again how I was struggling with this battle for my thoughts, and how it was preventing me from really, and finally, believing. As we talked, Don (who sometimes didn't actively participate in the dialogue because of his hearing disability) sighed, and said that God had led him to a scripture. As I now recall reading this with everyone that night, I am still struck with the wonder of the moment.

**The disciples came to him [Jesus] and asked, "Why do you speak to the people in parables?" He replied, "The knowledge of the secrets of the kingdom of heaven has been given to you, but not to them. Whoever has will be given more, and he will have an abundance. Whoever does not have, even what he has will be taken from him. This is why I speak to them in parables: "Though seeing, they do not see; though hearing, they do not hear or understand. In them is fulfilled the prophecy of Isaiah: 'You will be ever hearing but never understanding; you will be ever seeing but never perceiving. For this people's heart has become calloused; they hardly hear with their ears, and they have closed their eyes. Otherwise they might see with their eyes, hear with their ears, <u>understand with their hearts</u> and turn, and I would heal them" (Matthew 13: 10-15).**

At this point in my story, I want to say that I didn't really concentrate very much on the subject, or the significance, of parables in my own situation. I didn't know, at this time, just how important was Jesus' parable methodology in my own experiences with Scripture. It would turn out that His methodology to communicate truth would be, in fact, at the very core of my "spiritual insight" relationship with God. But, I don't want to give that away too soon. It would be incredibly exciting and encouraging in its time: God's time. What I did concentrate on, and what thrilled my spirit that evening when Don shared his gifted spiritual "hearing" through this scripture, was an answer to my ongoing battle of the mind with the enemy. It was also an explanation of the incredible, inner brokeness I was experiencing as God dealt with my significant relationships, my bitterness, my self-serving pride, and my past idolatries.

- **You will be ever hearing but never understanding; you will be ever seeing but never perceiving (Matthew 13:14).** I recognized my own frustration and weariness at not being able to fully receive, or fully believe, the amazing messages, pictures, and connections that were, evidently, being communicated to me in a supernaturally "coincidental" way. The longer the experiences continued, the greater and the more intense grew the mental debate with "reality" (the enemy). Each time my hope increased, I received a corresponding mental backlash from the enemy. This backlash not only dampened my newfound hope, but also increased the inner tension and self-criticism over my inadequate faith. Almost like breathing, I couldn't stop thinking my thoughts. Was all of this a phenomenon of faith or fantasy?

- **For this people's heart has become calloused; they hardly hear with their ears, and they have closed their eyes (Matthew 13:15a).** I almost started to weep when I read these words. **My heart** had become so "calloused", so hardened and bitter over the years. Cancer had first rendered me unable and then frozen in a struggle to "hear" or "see" past its hideous "reality." I began to understand why God was allowing me to experience cancer and the radical, painful **heartbreak** it had prompted in me through the past couple of months. I had often likened this heartbreak to a hammer or chisel violently breaking off huge pieces of petrified rock - like scar tissue from my heart, strata upon strata. Each blow exposed the raw, vulnerable, bleeding tissue underneath that was crying out for the life and healing of God. I was struck down by the realization that, without this **"rending" of my heart,** I wouldn't have possessed the ability to even comprehend what I had received thus far, let alone believe it with any certain faith. **(Remember Joel 2:12-27? I did.)** I also realized just how **intellectual** was my relationship with God. I had somehow forgotten my former life-changing experiences with Him, and had slowly relegated His reality and presence to the status of idealism in my life. The reality of God had been, regrettably, displaced to the mental realm of "godly" motivations and good intentions. This "form of godliness" was always subject to relativism and the ongoing "debate" with the reality of the world. I had forgotten that the power of His reality emanated from that treasured place at the very center of my being: my heart. God now had to break my heart to reach my center again. The best was still yet to come.

- **Otherwise they might see with their eyes, hear with their ears, understand with their hearts and turn, and I would heal them (Matthew 13:15b).** I did start to weep then, I think. The demon's battle for my mind was a clever and deadly diversionary tactic, a tactic designed to keep the reality of God, His healing, and His real power safely (for the demon) in the realm of ideas. As long as he was able to keep my understanding of God's amazing prophetic story at the mental level only, I would be engaged in the debate until it was too late for me. And not only too late to receive the healing that God was speaking about, but also, too late to communicate this transcendent message about cancer. Perhaps it would be too late for the realization that even my own salvation faith was just **"a house built on sand" (my mind only?) (Matthew 7:26).** Too late for anything that was truly life-giving, but just in time for death; earthly death, and possibly, even eternal death. God was showing me that, by breaking my heart, He was giving me the opportunity to "see," "hear," and "understand" **the real Truth of His Word** and of His presence in my life. By believing with a newly broken heart, my faith was in a protected place of sorts, away from the exhausting debate of the mind. As I weptand prayed about this incredible gift of insight, given through Don, I thanked God for unlocking this life-saving mystery to us. Connecting with His healing will actually begins with this "heart understanding." A new, heart-centered understanding helps us to finally turn away from the idol, and then it takes us to a place where God can really heal us.

At the end of the evening, I wrote these words in my notes: **"Satan has been attacking my faith in God's Word through my mind. Each time I think that I'm gaining assurance, the enemy reminds me that I have a deadly cancer, which can often re-occur. He's like clockwork. This Bible passage, which Don quoted, helped me to see that, for God's Word to be Truth, it had to be understood with the heart, not the head, lest it become just another part of the great debate of temporal "truth" with Satan. God has "spoken" to me through His Word about this illness and its reoccurrence. His Word is in direct opposition to what the enemy (and the world) is whispering to me daily. This scripture tells me that, without my "calloused" heart being changed, I would never be able to "understand" His Word to me (in my new heart) and receive His healing promise. I know that the mind battle will continue, but my heart is for God, and I pray for more faith to stand on His words to me." Amen...**

It's quite remarkable how God's timing, notwithstanding the whimsical, almost casual way in which believers utilize this term, became an object of greater certainty and wonder as my journey progressed. God's timing was truly remarkable, whether He was providing:

- direct answers to questions, prayed or not;
- more complex pieces to the puzzle regarding the larger, spiritual realm;
- loving assurances;
- greater clarity surrounding His personal healing words to me (and others);
- merciful and patient responses to my doubts and fears.

God must have known that the next few weeks were going to require a reservoir of supernatural experiences from which I might draw to keep my eyes focused on Him. My hope would need to be anchored in something other than my own physical resources.

# CHAPTER 22

# MURMURS IN THE DESERT

I was entering the halfway phase of my treatment. As I went each day to the clinic to wait, see, pray, and then receive radiation, I began to dwell more and more inside my "spirit bubble." As the routine of the clinic, the sights, sounds, smells, and faces became more familiar, these multi-sense images also became my main circle of awareness. They were my comrades on the "other side of the glass." They were my reason for prayer, for sorrow, for hope — my whole life, really. I don't want to say that the ongoing love and support of my family was lost on me; on the contrary. Unconsciously, my family was affording me the opportunity and the space to travel this road of "aloneness." They allowed me the journey without pressure, even if some their reactions were born out of perplexity as to exactly what I was experiencing. In spite of not completely understanding everything (how could we), I know that God was calling us back together as a family, albeit an unorthodox family. This whole experience with the Holy Spirit was a tad unorthodox anyway, don't you think? And, just as I became a card-carrying member of the "cancer club" (you really do carry a card), the club regulations dictated that treatment without side effects was really no treatment at all.

I will remind you, as I was reminded, of the irony of cancer treatment, that is, the irony of needing to manage the *side effects* of treatment quite separately and unrelated to managing the *disease* itself. It's a cruel irony and is part of the delusion of the idol. A cancer victim can be so overcome by the task of dealing with side effects, that a weird, separate battle, complete with options for victory or defeat, gets fought around these side effects. It can become so consuming that if the doctors or nurses tell you that you're "doing well" with the side effects, your desperation may translate this comment into a hope that you're, in fact, doing well against the actual disease. It's yet another opportunity for the cancer demon to discourage and demoralize you unto death. If the victim wants to believe that having success with the treatment's *side effects* somehow translates to *successful treatment*, then the victim's hope merely has a greater height to fall from once the real disease is evaluated. If the side effects are expectedly brutal, then the "pre-execution" torture is just more open, more terrifying (This is a provocative reason to reflect upon the psychological, pre-execution torture techniques employed by the Nazis against doomed Jewish prisoners). My own treatment side effects became the other focus of my life. They were the not-so-spiritual aspects of "the bubble."

- My taste buds finally, and completely, "collapsed." This is the only word that I can think of to describe what happened to my sense of taste. As we approached Christmas, a time of vivid memories and traditions of rich food and family, my body turned against me even more. The "strange" tastes of food (remember the nutmeg-flavored cheeseburger?), which had been simply undesirable before, gave way to tastes that were uniformly awful and even nauseating. I was warned, by the doctors, that taste changes would take place, which could mean absence of taste as well. But this was not an absence of taste, and was certainly not just "change." All food tasted vile — inedible.

- My throat started to become sore more slowly than they had predicted, but I could definitely feel more consistent pain. Another irony was that I had originally expected that my sore throat would prevent me from eating solid food. At this time, I was still mechanically able to eat, if I could find any food that didn't make me want to spit it out immediately. The lesson here was that, one way or the other, my eating days were (temporarily) over.

- The skin on my neck was finally showing signs of the radiation exposure over the last few weeks. I had never really sunburned in my life, yet the red soreness on both sides of my neck attested to the intensity of the "sunbeams" that I would face for another month. These sunburns would become real burns soon.

- I entered my second, scheduled week of chemotherapy during Christmas week; enough said. Merry Christmas.

I think that the reality of these side effects finally hit me on New Year's Day, 2003. I had already missed my extended family's Christmas dinner. It was a final admission of my total inability to stomach real food, as well as my veiled envy over others enjoying a normal, celebratory life. So, New Year's Day was like a knockout punch to a "game" but totally outclassed boxer.

In my family, New Year's Day was always the crowning culinary jewel of the year for an already food-obsessed clan. My late mother would lovingly toil for days to prepare a feast of all of our favorite foods. Each year on January 1st, along with a few privileged guests, we would consume vast quantities of these foods for, literally, the entire day. It was our way of welcoming the hope and the joy of a New Year. I was feeling the first, familiar hints of my chemo-induced nausea, in addition to the shocking destruction of my taste buds. My sisters sent a "care package" of New Year's goodies to the house. I was determined to take one last stab at the flavors of my youth, fueled by my memories of a once happy, bountiful life. (Do you get the feeling that food was another idol that God wanted to destroy?) I remember each tentative bite, of each different delicacy, and the overwhelming disappointment to my taste memories of what used to be my favorite foods. As I watched my children enthusiastically gobble up the care package, I dejectedly (really), even sorrowfully (really), turned to the new electric blender that Lori had purchased, in anticipation of my need for some nourishment. I began to prepare my first protein milkshake; the first of some 300 milkshakes that would serve as my "food" for the next three months. A couple of days later, at my weekly consultation with the doctor, I was told that, in many cases, the taste buds did not recover completely. And, since I was receiving radical (another fun cancer word) radiation therapy, I needed to be realistic about the possibility that my own recovery might only be partial. Like the icing on the cake (a cruel simile), this "compassion" from my doctor brought my morale to a new low. The thought of never being able to truly enjoy food again began to exert its discouraging weight against my fight for a healing faith. It is a weight that I strain to carry even today, months later, even having experienced God's gracious, healing love in so many ways. I am still recovering, and still, unsuccessfully, trying to enjoy food.

Perhaps it was the grace of God that I wasn't made aware of all of the eventual, treatment-induced consequences in early January 2003. The capitulation of my taste buds was probably all I could bear at that time. I know that I had no easy, man-made solution to look forward to. **All I could write in my notes about this present burden was that it was, "yet another thing to throw onto the mystery of God's mercy and grace."** The mystery was growing. I wasn't so sure if my faith was growing along with it.

It was about this time that God allowed me to begin an even more solitary portion of the journey. I was experiencing the combined effects of my taste bud trauma, the second chemotherapy, and the growing fatigue from treatment. On top of my personal burden was the daily witnessing of even greater suffering by other victims in treatment. Even as I was allowing these cancer realities to shade my life perspective, I was still struggling with the credibility of my own spiritual experiences of the past months. As remarkable and profound as these experiences had been, something in my darkened character kept me from fully accepting and fully believing the wonderful knowledge I was evidently receiving. God used yet another unique method to get my attention focused on this "issue du jour:" **the state of my weak faith, even in the face of persistent, loving communication from Him.**

I was in our bathroom, shaving. As I was prone to do out of habit, I was praying as I shaved. I was praying my normal "shopping list" prayer, though with a much greater sincerity born of adversity, but nevertheless, still quite routine. I had a habit of prefacing the **"healing for others" portion** of my prayer with the words **"Thank you Lord, for the truth of Your Word."** I would then proceed to pray for the healing and well being of friends and family. I had just spoken the aforementioned preface, When, very suddenly and abruptly, my head was filled with a deluge of very decisive and very "loud" words from a distinctly different source.

- **"Is it really the TRUTH, Fred?"**
- **"It cannot be only half-true."**
- **"Do YOU believe that it's truth, Fred?"**

- "If it is true, Fred, then why can't you believe it for yourself?"
- "YOU CANNOT PRAY FOR THESE PEOPLE IF IT ISN'T THE TRUTH!"

The last statement stabbed deeply into my heart, and I stood in front of the bathroom mirror, staring at my reflection. The voice was right. God was right. I could be standing right at the center of a monumental, biblical "rainstorm" of spiritual knowledge and healing mercy, complete with visions, voices, dreams, and miraculous *rhema* words from Scripture. Yet, if I did not, or could not believe the truth of the Word of God, this rainstorm of spiritual knowledge would mean nothing to me. It would have no power in my life. I would just become another victim of the idol. Even worse, perhaps, was the realization that not believing the Word for my own healing also meant not believing the Word for others. I was, therefore, guilty of hypocrisy by praying for them. Praying for healing, or anything else for that matter, when I could not truly believe that it would (or could) happen as the Word said it would, made me a hypocrite.

I further realized that I was being taken to places and concepts in the Word that were new and unfamiliar to me. These places and concepts had, heretofore, been objects of "suspended faith" for me. By suspended I mean that I had previously read them in the hope that I would never to have to confront them personally. In the healthy past, I could always comfortably view, from afar, the mystery of healing, the power of the Holy Spirit, and the issue of biblical inerrancy. These were "problematic" concepts that could be safely pondered to the end of my life. Like so many believers, I had felt vaguely secure in just (hopefully) getting right the whole "eternal salvation through Christ" thing. It was the most important thing, after all. There had been times when I even wondered if it was the only completely true thing in the Bible. Everything else in the Book, I reasoned, might be subject to the errors of time, the politics of religion or academia, and the misinterpretation of arcane languages, allegory and symbolism, or even the subjectivity of human authorship.

Yet, I couldn't avoid the notion that the voice was right. God was right. How could we anchor our lives in Him or depend on a God whose Word was flawed by human inconsistency or was only selectively or partially true? If the Word was not completely true, how could we know any of it was true? God was pushing me very hard to decide, even as He was working very hard (harder than I deserved) to show me His wonders. He even provided an "incentive plan" of sorts for me, to move to a place of greater faith for what He was sharing with me. He was moving me again, strategically speaking, to a place of heavy conviction, deep inside me, within my self-image.

Over the past many years I had succeeded in masking a damaged and darkened self-image with a more socially acceptable, confident, and "godly" external image. Everyone is aware of the emotional and spiritual scarring that takes place as a result of hidden resentment and sin. Without getting into my own numerous past sins, suffice it to say that Paul's famous, self-identification as the "chief of sinners" could have been subject to a trademark infringement dispute with me. I will admit to a life-long struggle with the whole concept of grace. Unmerited favor was a foreign concept to someone whose main life models (parents, admired relatives, and friends) were sincere, hard working "life earners." Many of these people were loving and encouraging achievers who lovingly encouraged performance and achievement in me. As I grew older and more aware of my accumulated affronts to God, the idea of grace took many years to grow credible roots. It took many more years for the idea to finally grow into an accepted and cherished gift that I could accept. My understanding of this gift would grow dramatically through the entire course of the journey, but in this particular case, **God brilliantly translated the fixation with my accumulated bad works into a unique reason to believe.** For this important time in my life, God gave me a fresh reason to believe the truth of what He was communicating to me, right now.

During this difficult "middle period" in my treatment, I wasn't getting the same distinct, encouraging connections or messages from the Lord. I wasn't receiving much through people, events, or even my daily open Bible reading. In fact, the growing stagnation of the "river" that had previously seemed to flow so freely from the Spirit was testing my faith in a new way. It wasn't just that the enemy was whispering his defeatist propaganda to me; that hadn't changed. What had changed was that God seemed to be communicating far less with me. What had seemed like a raging, rushing torrent of insight from deep inside the mystery of His Word was now a sluggish, spiritual eddy. It was difficult to accept, and more than a little scary. I found myself wondering if God had gotten "fed up" with my ongoing struggle to believe, even in the face of overwhelming, persistent evidence. I didn't realize that this fear was another expression of my habitual, performance-based, self-assessing personality. Throughout my life I hadn't laid up a whole lot of **"treasures in heaven" (Matthew 6:20),** but I had laid up a whole lot of rebellion and spiritual failure in my life. I wondered if His silence was simply a just response to another one of my spiritual failures: the failure to completely believe. My open Bible reading did, however, take me to a passage in Galatians about Abraham. God's recent "silence" had left me not expecting much.

Most believers who have had even limited exposure to "famous Bible quotes" have heard or read **Galatians 3:6**; I know that I had. **"Consider Abraham: He believed God, and it was credited to him as righteousness."** Although it provided only minor solace for the blockage of the "river,"

I did see this text (by the Spirit) in a completely different way than I had the previous times I had read it. Theological "correctness" notwithstanding, the words "believed" and "credited" became a kind of healing formula to my own accumulated "righteousness deficit." For some reason that only the Holy Spirit knows, I sensed that God was trying to encourage me to believe His recent words to me by appealing, quite brilliantly (as I had said), to my depleted self-image. It was both a present, and eternal, "win/win" grace offering to me. First, if I could grow in my belief, I would gain access to the wonderful healing and prophetic truths being shared with me. In addition, through this belief, I would receive a kind of bonus credit to my righteousness account in heaven. It was exciting to imagine how my sad shortage of righteous acts and my abundance of unrighteous acts, recorded somewhere in heaven, might be affected by this "credited righteousness." Did the text imply that if I could believe Him totally, then I would be seen as totally righteous? I wasn't exactly sure how this credit system worked, but the notion that believing Him carried with it this extra, eternal benefit did motivate me to seek more faith to believe. And for the first time in my life, I more fully understood how grace operated in the present and in the eternal.

Having left me with this extra bonus for believing Him, God then seemed to decide that this short, spiritual insight (Galatians 3:6) was sufficient to give me enough to ponder and pray about. It was sufficient to remind me that He was still pursuing me. It was sufficient to tell me that this was serious spiritual business. At some point, I had to realize that this was no longer an interesting, mental exercise for a healthy, inquiring believer. It was life or death itself.

Then, He let me wander in the desert for a while.

For the next two weeks or so, the side effects of the radiation treatment began to take over my every waking and sleeping moment. At the same time, my concentration on

God intensified. But, almost as if I was "trying too hard," my spontaneous and natural communication with Him seemed to disappear. Each day I would read my books, pray, reflect, and attempt my precious open Bible reading. But everything seemed to have deteriorated into a one-way conversation, spoken into silence and space. On the side-effect front, the radiation and chemotherapy had started to assault my body in a kind of "total war" mode.

- It seemed to take days longer to rise from the draining nausea of chemotherapy, and the radiation finally became a cruel flame, causing my throat to be so sore that even the milkshakes inflicted pain as the muscles contracted to swallow.
- The skin on the outside of my neck began to peel, exposing large areas of raw, suppurating soreness, as if I had been in some kind of unfortunate, incendiary accident.
- As my salivary glands, which were receiving much of the radiation, began to dysfunction, the irritation in my throat prompted the production of large amounts of a weird mucous and sputum discharge (pleasant description, I know). The discharge continuously accumulated in my throat. This accumulation had the effect of keeping me up most of the night, as it caused me to gag and choke enough to wake me up and keep me awake.
- I finally began another (remember my tonsillectomy?) long period (ten weeks, I think) of sleeping in a sitting position, to keep these foul secretions from accumulating in my throat. I finally began to get used to this arrangement, and in a twisted way, began to enjoy sleeping in this position. I wasn't sure that I would be able to sleep in a normal, prone position ever again.

- I continued to be despondent about the corruption and loss of my taste buds. Like some kind of masochist, I would from time to time attempt a bite of food. Often, I tried foods with flavors that I could remember vividly, fondly, and desperately. And each time, I would be more demoralized and terrified than the time before. All food had become truly vile, and I had only been drinking milkshakes (fortified by protein powder) for about three weeks. The future seemed to loom ahead forever, liquid and bleak.

- The effect of a totally liquid diet had its requisite impact on my digestion and **other bodily functions.** This impact was experienced frequently during the day and night (enough said). One ironic and cruel by-product of my milkshake diet was that the additional dairy intake caused even more throat mucous (see above: "sleeping in a sitting position"). Even the harmless milkshake had joined the cancer demon's supporting cast that both healed and tortured.

The accumulated burden of the side effects, combined with my constant struggle with fear, and then intensified (and dulled) by my fitful sleeping patterns, seemed to dominate my life and spirit. It was all I could do to hold on to the experiences of the previous weeks, and hang on to the faint notion that the Spirit was still walking with me. I hung on to the hope that God still wanted me to receive refreshment, knowledge, and healing. **During this two-week period in January, 2003, I made only a single, short entry in my notes, on January 17th: "Desert, Desert, Desert!!"**
I spent the better part of these two darkest weeks remembering what I had been shown. More importantly, I remembered the deep sense of wonder in my heart each time I had been given an insight or message by the Spirit. It was more than emotional; it was a "stirring" in my heart. Perhaps you

know what I mean. I kept on going back to the Matthew 13:10-15 passage about "understanding" with my heart and not my head. It encouraged me to continue believing with my heart, even if my head (and body) continued to struggle with doubt. My prayers started to contain words to the Lord about "receiving" into the protected place of my heart, which was now broken, laid bare, and willing to receive His truth. Even though the mental debate with the enemy continued, I began to slowly anchor myself in the message of the Matthew text. For truth to really be Truth, and for Truth's healing power to have its way, **Truth had to reside in the heart.** My body was in distress; kind of useless, really. My searching mind was continuously, and tediously, in conflict. But my heart, though struggling, was still spiritually hungry and reaching for God. And, as was His merciful way, He reached back for me, yet again.

# CHAPTER 23

# IT MUST BE GOD'S WILL

Here's another interesting connective device that God used to lead me back to the path of insight; **televangelism.** Each weekday morning, I would rise early to drive my youngest son to the train station, so he could catch the transit to his school. Sometimes, while I was waiting for him to get ready, I would turn on the television and watch a little of the programming on the 24-hour multi-faith channel. On one particular morning, while I was still in "the desert," I happened to catch a few, short minutes of a message from one of the American televangelists. He was quoting **Ecclesiastes 7:16-17:**

**Do not be overrighteous, neither be overwise – why destroy yourself? Do not be overwicked, and do not be a fool – _why die before your time_ [emphasis mine]?**

Although he wasn't talking about cancer necessarily, he was pointing out that **it was possible to die prematurely** before God's intended, ordained moment. In a way, this was like dying outside of, or apart from, God's **perfect** will. As I drove my son to the station, my mind was reeling again, and my heart was freshly encouraged, as I pondered the message of this text. I recalled my first spiritual impressions of the cancer establishment, where widespread suffering and death seemed so pervasive and indiscriminate. The term "God's will" seemed to be used so conveniently to explain the place of helplessness, defeat, and inevitability that so many victims were forced to accept. I remembered the notation that I had made in early December, some six weeks before, where I (reluctantly) wrote that I didn't believe it was always "God's will" that cancer victims suffer horribly and then die. Most of the time it's not easy to take a position on what God's will is or isn't. It's probably not even advisable. But, my "God's will" notation was most likely an example of a "heart understanding" that I had experienced in early December. It was an understanding that God was confirming with this scripture, read by a televangelist, weeks later.

I realized that, although God was God (sovereign, loving, powerful, and compassionate), we, the victims of the cancer demon, still had our part to play in the healing process or the dying process. And, this part had something to do with being "overrighteous" or "overwise," which could result in "self destruction" ("why destroy yourselves?"). I came to see the incredible, interwoven nature of this text in the accumulated learning of the journey so far.

- **"overrighteous"** — extremely religious types might have a tendency to passively accept the notion of death from cancer as an automatic demonstration of God's will. Or, at the other end of the spectrum, there are those ultra-spiritual types who believe that God's healing power is exclusively supernatural, and they sometimes resist the involvement or intervention of conventional medicine.
- **"overwise"** — whether religious or not, most people are very cynical, even critical, of the notion of God's

power in the question of literal healing or cure. They are the "realistic" ones; the ones who strongly advise against building on false hopes (for compassionate, even Christian reasons). Overwise believers avoid false hope by avoiding healing prayer, or by rationalizing the Bible as a limited, random factor in a possible, divine cancer healing. They, also, are among the first to acknowledge the spiritual healing intent of God, especially within the context of tested, scientific or psychological principles. The safe mode for Christian healing is often to keep it "spiritual" because it doesn't involve a requirement for physical evidence, such as disappearing tumors. This spiritual healing is called psychotherapy or counseling by overwise non-believers.

- I came to see that people could be **both** overrighteous and overwise. Often, through no fault of their own, they could be so scarred by their own experiences (with cancer, for instance) that finding Truth, then believing Truth, made it necessary for God to take them on a difficult path of discovery. I was on that path. To be overrighteous or overwise is to have a hardened or scarred heart that needs to be broken before it can believe with the right balance of righteousness and wisdom.

- A divinely broken heart can truly **"understand"** (**Matthew 13:15-16**). Such a heart prevents us from being a **"fool"** (**Ecclesiastes.7:17**).

- Being "overrighteous" was just as self-destructive as being **"overwicked"** (**Ecclesiastes7:17**). Wow, I thought.

- Remove the prefix "over" from the adjectives, and you have the words "righteous" and "wise." **This implied that demonstrating both qualities, in correct balance, would somehow prevent self-destruction,**

**wickedness, foolishness, and premature death.** I thought of Sandra Kennedy's teaching, and how she counseled the willing acceptance of conventional treatment (wise), in combination with believing God for supernatural treatment (righteous). What glorious encouragement that this journey was continuing and that my path was being somehow ordered by God!

- This passage in Ecclesiastes also helped confirm how we are often deceived into accepting the "reality" of cancer, even where the tragic outcome could be apart from God's will: **"why die before your time?"(Ecclesiastes7:17).**

A few days later, I would be led to another connection scripture; a connection within a connection, really. **Exodus 23:24-26** brought me back to the foundation of the teaching so far: *the danger of just surrendering to the idol.* At the same time, the text linked the false security of idolatry with the new Ecclesiastes insight of how we could become agents of our own premature death (meaning, at a time *not* of the Lord's ideal choosing).

This scripture is of the Lord speaking to Moses: **Do not bow down before their [Israel's enemies] gods or worship them or follow their practices. You must demolish them and break their sacred stones to pieces. Worship the Lord your God, and his blessing will be on your food and water. I will take away sickness from you, and none will miscarry or be barren in your land. *I will give you a full life span* [emphasis mine].**

- **"Do not bow down before their gods...worship... or follow"** — This was plain enough. Cancer victims, so often convinced that the idol is the truth, follow the idol to destruction.

- **"You must demolish them and break their sacred stones to pieces"** — This was new. It was a call to not only resist but to confront and destroy the idol. I wondered how we were supposed to attack when it seemed we were always on the defensive: weary, nauseated, mutilated, and afraid.
- **"Worship the Lord your God...I will take away sickness from you"** — Turning to the Lord with true recognition and worship was connected to a promise of healing. I wasn't ready to comprehend a **promise** from God, especially inside a disease that appeared to contain NO promises of any kind. The idol and the priests of the idol were constantly saying, "All we can truly promise is uncertainty."
- **"I will give you a full life span"** — Bowing to the idol (which is something **we** decide to do) short-changes us of the "full life span" planned by God. We can literally "die before our time."

Through this confrontation with the important truth inside these scriptures, God placed even greater pressure on me to believe. Mercifully, He also provided more believing faith through these same insights given by the Spirit. In a way, God wisely edified my faith from a new angle, **by giving me a determination not to "self destruct"** if I could help it. As I was receiving treatment, it was clear that the idol intended it to be my sole hope. I forced myself to divert faith energy from the actual treatment and to direct the energy toward an increased focus on God's sovereign management of the treatment. I tried to focus on His power over the physiological processes that I could see, or even those I could not see but could only imagine. It was an astute move by God to "jolt" me a little. He was showing me that, even if I could not **heal myself**, nor depend solely on conventional medicine to heal me, I could most certainly **destroy**

**myself.** The scripture suggested that I needed to look to God for "complete" healing, despite whatever way He wanted to accomplish it.

From a very young age, we are conditioned to expect positive results from medical treatment for our illnesses, and most of the time the results are not only positive, but tangible. If we have a cough, we take some cough medicine, and the cough goes away. If we have a wound of some kind, we bandage it or sew it up, and it heals with minimal scarring. With cancer treatment, tangible results are difficult to obtain, especially results that will provide the much-sought-after promise of a **cure.** If you distill down all the various, complex explanations and forms of the disease, the main reason for this difficulty with cure is that **cancer, as a disease, exists at cellular (and sub-cellular) levels.** The sub-cellular origins of the disease are virtually impossible to detect, trace, or contain in all the microscopic vastness of the human body. If you combine this minute, undetectable mechanism of the disease with the notion that **the "life" of cancer is actually spiritual** and unseen at its deepest foundation, you have a formula for disillusionment and defeat.

For some cancer victims, the struggle is intensified when the presence of this "deadly life" can be felt, or seen, or both, in some superficial way. Such was my struggle, as you might recall, with the outward evidence of my cancer being those infernal lumps under my chin and on my neck. Throughout the last few months, these lumps had become objects of my continual staring, checking, touching, probing, and measuring. I checked them in front of the bathroom mirror, while I was driving, while I was lying in bed (or sitting in bed, as the case may be), while I was anywhere. The lumps actually became somewhat of an idol unto themselves. Depending on their appearance, I would measure my progress in treatment, and at a deeper level, my progress in healing. At first, the lumps not only **did not** shrink but they actually got bigger, as an early response to radiation. Later on, the lumps did seem to get smaller, very, very gradually. But, by the time of my last week of treatment (some thirty-five radiation and two week-long chemotherapy sessions later) the lumps had, decidedly, not disappeared. My radiation doctor advised me that radiation did not work right away, due to the physiological processes which were affected: cell division and multiplication. Without getting too technical, radiation "kills" cancer cells, not by "burning" or "zapping" them instantly, but by messing up the DNA inside the cells. This radiation-induced disruption prevents cancer cells from reproducing, thus causing eventual cell death. This, of course, was the effect on irradiated **healthy** cells as well. But, who was counting cells anyway? This explained why my lumps had not shrunk away to nothing, even after two months of treatment. I would have to "wait and see" for at least another month or so; great.

If ever there was a time to reflect upon the "unseen battle" being fought inside my physical body and also somewhere in the spiritual realm, it was now. I had no choice but to turn my focus away from the hope of actually seeing immediate, tangible evidence of healing, directly from my treatment. I would have to direct my focus toward **waiting;** waiting for the clinical outcome, as well as for confirmation about what I had been spiritually receiving; waiting for God's "spin" on the battle with the cancer demon to be confirmed.

My last day of radiation finally arrived, but the journey through the desert continued. The side effects were still increasing, and as my throat and neck grew more raw, I viewed this long-awaited day as just the end of a chapter in a yet unwritten, unfinished story. I remember the enthusiasm of the radiation crew as the last appointment unfolded. There were comments about "how relieved I must have been that it was finally over," and, "what a "model patient" I had been. And, oh yes, "Good luck." I mean, what else could they say?

They had seen so much, and had so often been disappointed by the eventual outcome. As I walked out of the radiation unit, towards the day-patient room where I would receive my daily neck dressing, I felt the lumps on my neck once more. They were smaller, but not remarkably smaller. I forced my mind to think about God's "words" regarding this illness. I thought about what He had said, even specifically, about these lumps. I got my neck dressing applied, accompanied by the same enthusiastic wish of "good luck" from the nurse. I then proceeded to the wrap-up consultation with my doctor.

Although I will expand on this comment a little later in the story, my doctor's attitude in the previous couple of meetings had been almost "upbeat." He had never committed to anything definitively positive, on a clinical basis, but he was encouraging in tone and disposition. As he examined me and checked those ever-present, ever-frustrating lumps, his demeanor was reserved, even disquieting. He proceeded to tell me that he had given me the maximum radiation allowable (I knew that), and that we would have to wait at least a month to identify the full effect of the treatment. He "hoped" there would be significant shrinkage of the lumps, but it was difficult to predict how each lump, or even how each cell would react to the radiation. He didn't say that he was disappointed with the present status of the cancer, but I sensed that he was, a little.

This sense was verified when he began to discuss the possible contingency of radical neck surgery, or "neck dissection" as they call it (don't they dissect frogs and cadavers?!?). The surgery would be to completely remove the affected, as well as the suspect, lymph nodes. His description was thorough, vivid, and discouraging (again). It involved the necessity to "incise" (cut out) a significant length of neck tissue and muscle, and the possibility of some mobility loss and nerve damage in my right shoulder and upper arm (my guitar playing?). I tried to press him a little, asking him if he was saying that I would likely have to undergo surgery. He answered, carefully, that he could not predict surgery with certainty. But often, even smaller lumps didn't completely disappear under radiation, which often left no alternative but surgery. He just wanted to be "realistic" (there was the idol again) with me. He just wanted me to be "prepared" (the idol again). He didn't want me to have any "false hopes of complete cure" (and the temple band played on). He quoted some more statistics about the "control rate" for neck surgery, which I learned later has absolutely nothing to do with "survival rate" ("Welcome to my world," said the evil, grinning, leering idol).

I could feel myself deflating like a defective tire, when, mercifully, God brought to remembrance the first consultations: the statistics and the predictions for the future. **Isaiah 41** also came back to me, now three months later, with the same clarity and impact. **The "priests of the idol" were predicting my future, again.** God reminded me that I had been shown this before, and that it was even more important, now, for me to recognize the danger of idolatry. He reminded me of the absolute necessity for me to focus on Him for my future. We were heading for some kind of defining moment; the doctor knew it, I knew it, and God knew it. My challenge now was to wait for the next four weeks to pass, and when that moment would arrive.

# CHAPTER 24

# I'M NOT CRAZY
# (AT LEAST, NOT THE ONLY ONE)

Apart from my daily open Bible reading, I had cultivated the habit of going to the Christian bookstore every couple of weeks. I would pick up a few books to help me alter my focus, pass the time, and hopefully, better understand what God was doing with all of this. I would quietly slip into the aisles of the store and just browse the titles, cover notes, and authors. My choices would be guided more by intuition and "feel" than by any plan or persuasion. By mid-treatment, it was clear that God was guiding these choices as well. I admit to staying away from books about death, grief, or cancer. *(Note: There are always a few spiritually-themed books about cancer lining the shelves. They are mostly theo-practical guides to surviving or coping with cancer in the real world. I'm not saying that these books are not helpful to some people. They just weren't helpful for me)* I did end up reading a few books by pastors whose lives had been affected and changed by cancer. These books were less about cancer or healing than they were about changed lives. I read books about the Holy Spirit, divine healing, prayer, worship, prophecy, biographies, spiritual living, fearing God, doubting

God, surrendering to God — you name it. Throughout my three months of treatment, I probably read some forty books, all of which affected me in some way. All of them seemed to be mysteriously connected with the greater journey I was on. Sometimes, it would be just a few words or a sentence that seemed to speak directly to me. Sometimes it was a chapter, sometimes the entire book. In all cases, I was struck with just how powerfully God was "soaking" me in His awareness, His omnipresence, and His power. A number of times in this literary journey, I would be led to a place of spiritual connection or insight that would rival any of my other experiences with Scripture, people, or dreams. *(Note: I think I briefly mentioned [without fully explaining] one of these connections, in reference to my first articulated exposure to the "cancer idol" image: Hope's powerful testimony. It involved the discovery of a close paraphrase of my own written notation of this event in a book on healing authored by an American Lutheran pastor. This discovery was some two months after my notation was recorded. I will eventually recount this discovery to you when my story reaches that moment, chronologically.)*

One key example of God's amazing commitment to my "literary education" occurred on one of these trips to the bookstore, a day or so after my last treatment. As I was gazing at one of the rows of books, the title *He Still Speaks Today* (YWAM Publishing House, c. 1997) seemed to jump out at me. This was one of the ways I seemed to be drawn to the "right" book choices. I drew the thin paperback off the shelf and didn't immediately recognize the name of the author, **John Sherrill**, as being very significant to me. But, as I read the brief cover notes on the back of the book, my heart started doing that familiar "stirring" thing again, as it had so often over these last few months. **For one thing, it turned out that John Sherrill, along with his wife Elizabeth, had co-written two books which, many years before, had** become significant "life books" for me: *The Cross and the Switchblade* (co-written with Rev. David Wilkerson) and *The Hiding Place* (co-written with Corrie ten Boom). I had read these books so long ago that I had forgotten their common authorship. More importantly, as I read the brief description on the book cover, my knees felt weak as I read the following words:

- "John Sherrill did not expect God to use the Bible to speak to him personally, but He did!"
- "Lacking a compass to (stay close to the Word)... he nonetheless charged forward...headlong into an amazing adventure with the Bible."
- "To John's astonishment, the Scriptures took on new meaning as they truly became the Living Word of God to him."
- "Your God is not silent....He still speaks through Scripture."
- "It's easy to forget the reality of God's presence, and His desire for your companionship, His readiness to help you in every situation."
- "Can God actually speak to me from the Bible?"

As I read these words, I knew that God was trying to confirm His personal involvement in my own scriptural experiences of the past few months. And even though, upon reading the book, some of the details of Sherrill's "Bible dialogue" with God were somewhat different than mine, **the essentials of the relationship were amazingly similar.** Especially similar were the personal *rhema* insights relevant to Sherrill's own life circumstances and faith position. These insights were "embedded" or "hidden" by the Spirit inside the literal words of the various texts. Just like me, Sherrill read Scripture literally, and then, simultaneously connected with a deeper insight or picture that God intended specifically for him: *rhema*. I don't need to tell you how encouraging the discovery of this book was for me, just at the time when I needed new encouragement. The aggravating and painful side effects of my treatment were beginning to "peak." I was standing just at the front entrance of the long, four-week "corridor" leading to the clinical results of the treatment.

Oh, one last thing: I said my heart was stirring as I realized that God's hand was in the discovery of this book. That stirring became a whirlpool and then a tidal wave when, a few days later, I reached the part in the story where (almost as a footnote, really) **John Sherrill described his own journey with cancer — cancer of the head and neck, complete with swollen lymph nodes on his neck — cancer healed by the power and the love of God. Praise Him forever.**

# CHAPTER 25

# DARK NIGHTS OF THE SOUL

B y the end of my treatment cycle, the severity of my side effects had committed me, indefinitely, to a strange and new life routine.

-   Ingesting all of the nourishment for my body in liquid (supplement or milkshake) form.
-   Popping painkillers on a schedule to coincide with my "meals" so my throat could bear the discomfort of swallowing the liquid.
-   Wearing white gauze dressings around my burned, raw neck that looked a little like a "dickie" from the 1970s. I tried to "complement the look" with other clothing whenever I had to venture out into the world. I'm not kidding. I don't know if I really fooled anyone.
-   Resting and napping frequently during the day. This was caused, in part, by the fitful, restive, night sleeping patterns of one who has to sit up (in an easy chair moved to a corner of our bedroom) so as not to gag on mucous.

- Getting up frequently, day and night, to expel mucous as well as other bodily excretions caused by this routine (enough said, again).

Even as this routine, which would carry on for the next two months or so, was difficult to bear in one way, in another way, God used these long nights of waking and sleeping to communicate with me in a fresh manner. Often, when I would be lying (oops, sitting) awake at 3:00 AM or 4:00 AM, with Lori sleeping quietly in the bed across the room, I would experience a rich time of reflection, prayer, and communion with God. His quiet, atmospheric presence would sometimes fill the darkened space and just surround me. At other times, I could sense deeper direction to my thoughts and feelings connected to the overall journey. In some ways I would look forward to this time of wakeful silence and yes, peace. Now, in this silence, I was not being so easily overwhelmed with thoughts of defeat and fear. Perhaps my faith was growing stronger than I thought. This growth was important, since, in the absence of any further practical treatment for the disease, I now had nothing but faith and the memory of my incredible experiences to "lean" on as I pondered the future and my fate.

I remember lying awake on one of the more miserable of these nights. I was feeling my feelings. My spirit was being crushed a little in the silence and the darkness, and my throat was very sore. I was despairing in my memories of food, and my stomach was gurgling like a milkshake-filled jacuzzi. My heart was overflowing with longing, and I cried out in my spirit, "God, can You restore this damaged, decrepit body of mine?" Almost spontaneously, my head was filled with the answering words, "Remember, I am the One who resurrects dead flesh!" I guess damage and decrepitude are no "big whoop" for God. I was encouraged and comforted. I went to sleep; for a while, anyway.

On yet another late night, when the house was dark and quiet, my reflections were led back to some earlier thoughts that I had entertained about the nature of the biblical adversary, Assyria. I thought about the nation as an image of the cancer stronghold. And, I thought about the personality or character of the King of Assyria, as an image of the spirit of cancer. All the descriptive words I had thought of (arrogant, powerful, prideful, purposeful, cruel, deceptive, god-like) brought me back to **a suspicious "link." It was a link between these spiritual images of Assyria (inside Isaiah and 2 Kings) and the best known characteristics of the ultimate evil one, Lucifer.** Again, it was as if God was waiting until this particular moment to fill my heart with the confirmation that this "link" was in fact a real relationship. This relationship was between the spiritual picture of cancer, as revealed to me in the scriptures about Assyria (or the Midianites), and the eternal foundations of evil, as revealed in the person of Lucifer, the enemy. Although I didn't take the time that night to find the scriptural references, I remembered enough of the story of Lucifer's pride and arrogance. Especially interesting were the connections to Lucifer's own rebellion, even after being elevated to the highest angelic status (raised up like Assyria, by God Himself). It was this rebellion which ultimately caused his expulsion from heaven. All these very same characteristics had been exhibited by those cruel, idolatrous, conquering Assyrian hordes.

At the same moment, another overwhelming image entered my mind. It was an image of Jesus cursing the fig tree. Simultaneously, I had a memory of my wife Lori seeing a prayer image, early in the journey, of my cancer being "choked off at the root." It was like a light turning on suddenly in my darkened bedroom. **I realized why cancer must be fought on both a clinical and spiritual level in order to enable God's healing will to be fully realized. In Mark 11:20,** the disciples discovered that the fig tree, cursed by Jesus, had **"withered from the roots."** The fig tree had no chance to grow back, because the unseen part of the tree — the roots below ground which provide essential nourishment — had also been destroyed. I saw so clearly, in the darkness of the night, that the tree was a picture of the physical disease. The "tree" could be cut down or cut off, it could be burned, but its life would still be present underground, threatening to send up new shoots, new growth. **The roots of the tree represented the spirit, the real (evil) life of the tree. This evil life couldn't be killed or cast out by man, but only by Jesus Himself, with a Word spoken from His mouth,** and just as Lucifer had been cast out of heaven with a word spoken by God Himself, somewhere in time eternal.

This period of time, just after the completion of my treatment and just before I was to find out the status of my illness, was probably the most difficult part of the journey thus far. In addition to struggling with the physical ramifications of treatment (I won't burden you with yet another commentary on side effects), the psychological battle with the enemy just seemed to rage on, day after weary day. There was a difference, however, in the "game of inches" that this battle had become. I was no longer losing ground an inch at a time. Nor was I just "trading blows" with the demon in a spiritual stalemate. For the first time, I sensed that my faith was **growing** by inches. It seemed that this growth was from the foundation of "noncoincidental coincidences" and from the "good roots" that God had been so faithfully planting in my broken heart from the beginning of the journey. My faith was actually becoming more real as a result of seeing "reality" in this supernaturally new way.

I do remember another lonely night around this time, when I was feeling particularly sorry for myself. I was angry, bitter, and resentful about the physical ordeal, the lack of control, the complete uncertainty about the future, and having to give up so much of my life (even though I knew that much of my life had been wrong-hearted anyway). I wasn't openly complaining to God, but He knew what was in my heart that night. As I continued in my open Bible reading, I was brought to my senses, again, through the leading and the conviction of the Holy Spirit. I was rather absently, even with a little irritation, turning the pages of my Bible, searching through the Psalms. I was scanning the first few words of each selection, wondering if I would be compelled to stop at any time. I was, perhaps, a little perturbed that a connection didn't seem to be "happening" as spontaneously as before. After a while, I got tired of just scanning the pages, and decided, when I reached **Psalm 66**, that I would just read this particular Psalm in its entirety and then move on to another section of the Bible. As I read Psalm 66, the beginning verses were typical worship prose about a God who reigns over a joyous and grateful creation.

- **Shout with joy to God, all the earth! Sing the glory of his name; make his praise glorious! Say to God, "How awesome are your deeds!" (Psalm 66:1-3)** The next six verses just seemed to go on and on with this theme of power, glory, and joy, and I felt even more miserable as I pictured myself on the "wrong side" of this joy. At the same time, I was feeling even more ungrateful and petty despite all that God had been sharing with me over the last few months.

I was about to quit on this Psalm. It would be much better to dive into the sympathetic darkness of one of David's compositions about illness, depression, and desperation. Then, just as my self-pity and ingratitude reached its peak, I read these words:

- **He has preserved our lives and kept our feet from slipping (Psalm 66:9).** This one verse was the Spirit's "sword" which pierced my heart, and I stopped breathing for a second. Then I started "bleeding" from the wound, weeping tears of conviction. God was "preserving my life" from a fate of eternal torment and misery. He didn't have to do this. He could have just let me live on in my bitterness, delusion, and idolatry. He could have allowed me to perish, physically, at the foot of the cancer idol. He could have, perhaps, allowed me to suffer forever, spiritually, because of my hardened, unbelieving heart. I remember thinking, quite involuntarily, that this whole experience with cancer (which might include death), was a justifiable trial to endure when compared to the larger gift that He was giving me. It was the gift of showing Himself to me, in this way, and then saving me for heaven. This must have been the Holy Spirit's doing, because it was so uncharacteristic of me to actually think eternally (who really wants to think about death) in preference to the world that I could see and wanted so desperately to hold on to. The Holy Spirit was clearly speaking from deep inside of me, because the "natural" Fred still wanted desperately to live.

- **For you, O God, tested us; you refined us like silver. You brought us into prison and laid burdens on our backs. You let men ride over our heads; we went through fire and water, but you brought us to a place of abundance. (Psalm 66:10-12)** I was very emotional now, as I saw myself inside that prison. It was a prison defined by cancer, but a prison still under God's wardenship. He had admitted me to this prison (as I had always believed), but it was more like "protective custody" designed to "preserve" my life for Him. The images of "men riding over our heads" resonated with my history of doctors, technicians, and clamped-down radiation masks. The "fire and water" spoke of my radiation and chemo-therapy. My heart, though broken by conviction, was also comforted and encouraged by this prison image. Because, if He put me in this prison, it was not a place of execution, but a place of discipline and teaching ... a place of enforced waiting ... waiting to be rehabilitated, paroled, and finally, "brought ... to a place of abundance."

From that time on, I never found it very easy to be resentful of God for my illness (even if I still couldn't thank Him for it). The "prisoner" image would stay with me and even bless me with greater understanding later on (... as the "prisoner," even now, writes these words from his "cell").

# CHAPTER 26

# THE QUESTION OF GRACE

I have failed to mention a particular detail, and I feel the time is appropriate to do so, especially after all the complaining regarding my treatment side effects. The overdue detail is that I had gained an ongoing sense, in spite of the obvious struggles, that God was demonstrating a special grace to me in the severity and duration of those side effects. The reason that I say this is really threefold:

- First, as each side effect was monitored and evaluated weekly by the doctors and nurses, I received a fairly consistent flow of comments that indicated surprise, and even a little puzzlement, as to why I was not more affected. Why was I not more tired? Why was my throat not more sore than it was? (They even prescribe morphine syrup and IV nourishment for some patients.) Why was my neck, though burned quite severely, healing so quickly? Why was my weight actually increasing? (I was able to thank God for the milkshakes.) I concentrated on remembering that these "positive" comments were just in reference to the side effects and not the real disease. Nevertheless, everyone seemed a little perplexed as to why my side effects seemed less severe than expected.

-   Second, my daily trips to the cancer clinic exposed me to the entire spectrum of patients, treatments, and side effects. Each day, as I have described earlier in the notes, I observed and absorbed images of suffering, perseverance, courage, and sadness that will stay with me forever. As I sat among my "brothers and sisters," locked in the struggle with the idol, I knew that somehow God was helping me stand on the edge of the abyss of despair. He was enabling me to understand its depth while still holding me and keeping me from falling in.

-   Third, this sense of grace, of being somehow "shielded" from the worst of the treatment side effects, brought me to a place of questioning about grace. This questioning began sometime in December 2002 as the side effects began, and continued daily (really) until early February 2003. It was in February that God, knowing that this question about grace was being asked again and again, finally showed me that He was ready to answer. But, only in His way, in His time.

Like I said, this question about God's grace in my treatment experience haunted me right from the beginning. I knew that many people were praying for me, and yet this seemed an incomplete explanation, especially as I witnessed the terrible suffering of so many other patients at the clinic. Many of them had sincere intercessors praying for them as well. "The question" was really several questions:

-   Why me?
-   How were my circumstances different from the others?
-   Who deserved it more, or less for that matter?

It was clear that these questions about side effects were just the "warm-up act" to the same big, lingering questions about the disease itself. In my Bible reading, I had studied Jesus' healing ministry, which had birthed a growing conviction about God's general healing will for all of us. However, God's other "teaching," shared with me over the last months, had proven that there were other variables in the healing journey. For example, I was coming to an understanding of the role that our own idolatry would play in this journey. But there was still the ever-present principle of God simply being God. So, even if we turned from every idol that we could identify, this did not establish any kind of "bargain" or "formula" that God was bound to follow, honor, or otherwise capitulate to. I mean, He was perfect and sovereign; we were not. It was an obvious mistake to believe that we could gather an irrefutable body of evidence, justifying our case for healing, and receive some guaranteed, programmed response from God. I'm not trying to get into the whole (endlessly argued) controversy about the "name it and claim it" view of God as "the supernatural vending machine." However, I will say that God's will to heal became **THE** key principle on which I anchored my faith and hope. Yet, knowing that my understanding of His will was so limited by my own humanness, I never forgot Who would ultimately define the principle. It's like knowing that the law of gravity exists, generally, but not completely understanding how mass, weight, composition, and external conditions will affect how gravity works on specific objects (I think).

Anyway, as I continually asked these questions about grace, my open Bible reading time afforded God the opportunity to answer with precision, clarity, and power. I was leafing through the **New Testament** this time, and as I moved through the book of Romans, my eyes rested on the heading **"God's Sovereign Choice" (Romans 9).** You *know* that I had to stop here, and as I scanned the verses of this chapter, I reached the passage that I believe was the planned destination.

- **Not only that, but Rebekah's children [Jacob and Esau] had one and the same father, our father Isaac. Yet, before the twins were born or had done anything good or bad – in order that <u>God's purpose in election</u> might stand: not by works but by him who calls – she was told, "The older will serve the younger" (Romans 9:10-13).** Election, Election, Election. Before birth, before any deed, good or bad. God just being God. God making a decision, not because of works, but through a "calling." A calling that He bestows on an individual, even an individual sinner. The light was coming on again.
- **What then shall we say? Is God unjust? Not at all! For he says to Moses, "I will have mercy on whom I have mercy, and I will have compassion on whom I have compassion." It does not, therefore, depend on man's desire or effort, but on God's mercy (Romans 9:14-16).** God was being merciful to me, in spite of my desires or efforts, both past (thanks to God for "overlooking" them) and present (my feeble, fragile faith).
- **For the Scripture says to Pharoah: "I raised you up for this very purpose, that I might display my power in you and that my name might be proclaimed in all the earth" (Romans 9:17).** I am quietly substituting the name "Fred" for "Pharoah." Am I proclaiming His power now?
- **But who are you, O man, to talk back to God? Shall what is formed say to him who formed it, "Why did you make me like this?" Does not the potter have the right to make out of the same lump of clay some pottery for noble purposes and**

**some for common use? (Romans 9:20-21)** God was saying to me, "OK, are we clear now? Stop asking 'Why?' Just accept the grace and the wisdom that I am sharing with you now. I have a purpose for you that I decided upon before you were born, before your sins. I knew you that you would be (completely) undeserving of this present grace. Aren't you glad that this part has nothing to do with your works?"

I was glad. I was also encouraged by this new knowledge which confirmed that I was still walking on the road of insight with the Spirit of God. I was encouraged by the grace that God was confirming with these words. I was also allowing myself to look further, or deeper, at the hope (or hint, at least) of "purpose" which had been mentioned here as well.

The word "purpose" blessed my heart, and I thought about the wonder (and fear) that Gideon must have felt at being asked to be God's instrument of deliverance from the Midianites. I thought about the broad canvas being painted (beyond my own illness) depicting God's battle with the stronghold of cancer. I let my mind go, just for a moment, wondering if there was going to be a purpose for me. And, just as quickly, as my head started spinning with the possibility, I pulled back from the presumption. And, I just pondered the grace part again. Then, I thought about Jim, the man who didn't even ask for his brain tumor to be healed. He just happened to be "somewhere in the crowd" when Jesus' healing will was brought to bear on him anyway. I remembered feeling, then, somewhat uncomfortable, even a little "shortchanged" by Jim's story of healing. But now, I realized that God wanted me to remember Jim's story in this new light of understanding. It wasn't that He was disregarding my efforts to seek Him. It wasn't that my decision to turn from idolatry wasn't important. The new understanding helped me to realize that God understood my limitations; in knowledge, strength, and faith. God knew that I was trying to fulfill my part of the relationship despite all my human weaknesses. He was also showing me that, in spite of my failures, He could still choose me, shield me from hopelessness, and even heal me for His own reasons (election). Only God could "complete" this process of relationship. I stopped asking "Why?" that very night.

# CHAPTER 27

# BAND OF SURVIVORS

This period of new enlightenment, which began as I emerged from earthly treatment as well as my spiritual desert, was to continue at an accelerated pace over the next few weeks. God was preparing me for the trials of waiting, watching, and finally, facing my clinical condition to be "unveiled" at the beginning of March 2003 (where did all the time go, Lord?). In spite of the obvious faith requirements for absorbing and believing what I was being shown, I was mostly blown away by the sense of God's mercy and patience toward me. A huge example of this patience was the way He supported the faith journey by continuing to appeal to my mind (darkened though it was), my common sense, and even my logic.

The connections or "common threads" inside the incredible story God was telling me was like being in some kind of "living tapestry." This "tapestry" was continually being woven into a larger cloth. At the same time, the Weaver was adding new threads to selected portions of the "tapestry" for depth, color, and substance. The Holy Spirit was using so many amazing, supernatural media with which to "educate" me, that the name "Counselor" took on new meaning for me.

- The scriptural insights continued to develop into "parallel" stories. They were images of my own circumstances, as well as something more general or "globally" significant. I was still hesitant to use the word "prophetic," but there was no doubt that God wanted to communicate His grace to me in a very multi-dimensional way. First, there was a "prophetic" quality in the manner which specific aspects of my situation were being identified and addressed by His "words." At the same time, the images of the cancer stronghold, the cancer idol, and the eternal story of warfare were always present. These images acted as a kind of "calling" to something more purposeful, more "prophetic" if you will (there, I've just used the word twice).
- Often through the journey, God would use these "common threads" to confirm or reinforce something He had already shared, but also to create completely new insights. These new insights would re-direct or even establish an important new path on the journey. Now was to be such a time. It was God's perfect timing, again.

You might recall that **2 Kings 18 and 19** had provided some of the first most vivid and most descriptive pictures of the spiritual stronghold of cancer. (This portion of Scripture was first encountered in November 2002, over two months previous.) This passage had deeply encouraged me.

- First, through its images of God's awakening to the demon's arrogance and cruelty.
- Then, through His protection of a besieged people.
- And finally, through His powerful victory over the hordes of the enemy.

One key reference in the 2 Kings 19 passage had stayed with me, lingering in my heart for the past two months. It was a unique reference, one which had not been specifically addressed since that time: **"For out of Jerusalem will come a remnant, and out of Mount Zion a band of survivors" (2 Kings 19:31).** I can still remember thinking, as I read this verse, that God was suggesting that this journey of truth was being traveled by others, or one day *would be* traveled by others. He meant for His healing message to be heard and believed by all those who could truly **"understand with their hearts" (Matthew 13:15). Could they be "a remnant," perhaps?** I also remember being moved by the use of the term "band of survivors." This expression connected the text to the identity of cancer. It suggested that the whole point of the journey was to increase the number of cancer survivors, which, praise God, seemed to include me. The word "remnant" would stay with me, although I didn't really understand its biblical significance until later. God used the word "remnant" to lead me on that important new path that I spoke of a few sentences ago.

My previous experience with Romans 9, involving the concept of "election," whetted my appetite to stay in that book. So, the very next night, I continued my open Bible reading there. A couple of pages after my Chapter 9 starting point, my eyes came to rest on the heading **"The Remnant of Israel" (Romans 11).** You know that this was too good to pass up. I wasn't disappointed either.

- **God did not reject his people, whom he foreknew (Romans 11:2a).** There was that reference to election ("foreknew"). Was it a common thread, starting a new section to the tapestry?
- **Don't you know what the Scripture says in the passage about Elijah – how he appealed to God against Israel: "Lord, they have killed your prophets**

**and torn down your altars; I am the only one left, and they are trying to kill me" (Romans 11:2b-3).** No, I didn't really know what "the Scripture says in the passage about Elijah." I did recall that he was a prophet, and that he was one of just two people in history who had been taken up to heaven without dying first. I also had a vague recollection of his involvement with the prophets of Baal, but I could not remember the exact story around it. "Israel," I imagined, was an idolatrous nation, and the image of the idolaters trying to kill Elijah resonated into my situation. "I am the only one left" reminded me of how alone I felt in this journey, and especially alone (save for Lori, Warren, Laurie Lee, Hope, and Don) in this unique, spiritual picture that God was painting. I mean, who else might believe me?

- **And what was God's answer to him? "I have reserved for myself seven thousand who have not bowed the knee to Baal. So too, at the present time there is <u>a remnant chosen by grace.</u> And if by grace, then it is no longer by works; if it were, then grace would no longer be grace (Romans 11:4-6).** A remnant "who have not bowed the knee" to the idol (Baal, cancer, whatever); a remnant "chosen by grace." This phrase illuminated the journey like a new streetlight over a previously dark alley. How could we survive cancer if we believed solely in the earthly "reality" that the idol represented? How could we become the "remnant" or "band of survivors" unless we recognized the lies of the idol and then turned back toward God? How could we "understand" the Truth that was offered about the idol if our hearts were hardened and our minds darkened? All these questions were a path leading backward to the very first insight I had experienced at the beginning of the journey. I realized that this first insight, in fact the entire journey, would not have been possible if my heart had not been broken sufficiently. Broken, so that I might "understand" the answers to those important questions. This initial breaking of my hardened heart (prompted by my illness) was not of my choosing (or a result of my "works"). It was a loving act of grace from a loving God, who was merely "helping" me **to "understand" the path of the "remnant."** He was showing me how to join the "band of survivors," and how His truth could turn the remnant into an army or even a nation. Without this gracious gift of "understanding" in the depths of a God-broken heart, there would be no Fred, nor any chance to join the "remnant chosen by grace."

# CHAPTER 28

# AND THEN, THERE WAS ELIJAH

Like I've said, I didn't know very much about Elijah at that time. In a superficial way, I did remember that he was a prophet, that he had been translated to heaven without first dying, and that he had somehow been involved in a confrontation with Baal worshippers. The reference to Elijah in Romans 11 was new to me, but I had learned enough about these new, scriptural connections that there was no doubt in my mind that I had to read about him somewhere in the Bible. I looked up "Elijah" in my concordance and noted that the book of 1 Kings contained the majority of the references, so I turned to this new place in my Bible. I began to read **Elijah's story in 1 Kings 17,** reading through the whole course of the chapter and into the next. While reading, I gained a better sense of the supernatural nature of his ministry, as well the tension that existed between the powerful Baal worshipping monarchs, Ahab and Jezebel, and the dwindling followers of the true God.

**By the beginning of 1 Kings 18,** it was clear that some kind of decisive confrontation was developing between the two factions. The Baal "camp" clearly held more of the "intimidation cards" in the high stakes game that was unfolding. Many of the faithful prophets of God had already been killed by Ahab and Jezebel (I remembered this from Romans 11). These two "champions of the idol" might have completed their genocidal plan, but God visited a severe drought, followed by a famine, upon their kingdom. Elijah was raised up by God to be His representative and spiritual "champion" in the decisive confrontation to come. Elijah was first instructed to present himself to Ahab, armed with a prophecy about the future — a much-needed rainstorm. This command for Elijah to appear before the enemy Ahab caused great dismay in one of the few remaining Israelites faithful to God. His name was Obadiah, who just happened to be Ahab's senior palace servant. Obadiah reluctantly, and fearfully, arranged the first face-to-face discussion between Ahab and Elijah. Elijah had been instructed to demand a grand "summit meeting" on Mount Carmel. This meeting would be attended by Elijah, Ahab, 450 prophets of Baal, and 400 prophets of Asherah (a "sister" god to Baal). There would also be in attendance an unknown multitude of witnesses identified in the text simply as "the people" (there must have been a substantial number of interested onlookers for such an epic event). This gathering at Mount Carmel was to become a defining moment in the generations-old conflict between God and Man's idolatry.

God chose to prosecute this battle in a most dramatic fashion. First, Elijah instructed the people to obtain two bulls and then to erect two sacrificial altars, side by side. There was to be one altar for Baal and one altar for God. He then gave the prophets of Baal the first opportunity to make their sacrifice, with one key stipulation. They were not to light a fire in order to burn the bull upon the altar, but instead, they were to call upon Baal to light the fire supernaturally. The next few verses described the frenzied efforts of all 450 prophets of Baal. They desperately spent themselves, dancing around their altar, loudly crying out to their pagan god, even mutilating themselves with swords and spears. This intense display went on for approximately eight hours (the text says morning till evening), all in the hope of receiving supernatural fire from their god. No such fire resulted. The bull sacrifice to Baal remained untouched in the sight of all the onlookers.

Then, Elijah stepped forward and began giving instructions to the people for the sacrifice to the true God. In addition to laying the bull upon the other altar, he commanded that a deep trench be dug around the perimeter of the altar. He then instructed that large jars of water be poured over the bull and the altar. But, as if this was not enough of a "starting handicap" for God, Elijah had the people repeat this procedure twice more, so that the water overflowed the altar and even filled the surrounding trench.

- Then, when all this had been done, Elijah prayed these words: **"O Lord, God of Abraham, Isaac, and Israel, let it be known today that you are God in Israel and that I am your servant and have done all these things at your command. Answer me, O Lord, answer me, so these people will know that you, O Lord, are God, and that you are turning their hearts back again"** (1 Kings 18:36-37).
- When Elijah had finished his prayer, **"Then the fire of the Lord fell and burned up the sacrifice, the wood, the stones and the soil, and also licked up the water in the trench. When all the people saw this, they fell prostrate and cried, 'The Lord – he is God! The Lord – he is God!'"** (1 Kings 18:38-39)
- Then, while this "shock and awe" accompanying God's incredible display of power was still fresh among the people, **"Elijah commanded them, 'Seize the prophets of Baal. Don't let anyone get away!' They seized them, and Elijah had them brought**

**down to the Kishon Valley and slaughtered there"**
**(1 Kings 18:40).**

It's an incredible story, right? This is a classic confronta-tion between the power of God and the power of an idol. No contest; not even close. God first sees us being terrorized, tortured, and killed by demonic forces. Then He sets up a decisive showdown in the sight of all the intimidated victims and bystanders. And then, He "conquers the conquerors" with devastating, lethal force. This story resonated loudly with all the other stories, scriptures, and pictures that I had received on the journey.

Yet, it wasn't the story itself that God used to visit His own "shock and awe" upon me (although Elijah's story would become incredibly important soon enough). **God first prompted me to read about Elijah to force a similar confrontation, deep inside my heart. He was finally about to tell me that it was time to "grow up" in my own faith.** He had been so faithful, so relentless, so patient, and even so repetitive that I often pictured Him sitting in heaven, wondering when I was *finally* going to "get it." So, as the appointed time for my treatment results approached, as the "moment of (eternal) truth" approached, I believe that God had decided to confront **me**. He had decided to confront my "conditional" faith directly. This was the real, initial purpose of the Elijah connection, and the reason that I have merely paraphrased and not really explained the whole text as I have done with previous scriptures. Because, on this first reading of the story, one to which I would return many times, I did not receive a spontaneous, spiritual picture as I read the words. That, evidently, was not God's first intent. **His purpose, I believe, was to speak to me directly**, even bluntly, about life and death. He was speaking to me **about what and Who I would choose to believe** as my personal battle was fought and decided. He had done so much to show me the Truth beyond the earthly reality of the cancer idol. He had communicated the availability of hope and healing, not just for me, but for a whole "band of survivors" as yet unidentified. Up to now, it had been convenient and safe to discuss my experiences as amazing, "noncoincidental coincidences." My initial reaction to these experiences had always been conviction and wonder, but the follow-up reaction had invariably been doubt and reason. The whole experience was continually colored by a lingering fear of the world's "reality." **But, Truth is not personal Truth until it is believed and acted upon.** So now, He was talking directly to me, about me. My heart jumped, my breathing stopped, as I could almost hear God challenging me through **Elijah's words to the people in 1 Kings 18:21, 24.**

How long will you waver between two opinions? If the Lord is God, follow him; but if Baal is God, follow him." **But the people said nothing. Then you call on the name of your god (Baal), and I will call on the name of the Lord. The god who answers by fire – he is God.**

This passage is all that I remember reading that night (according to my notes made at the time), although I must have read the whole story that I just paraphrased. I sat for quite awhile, stunned by the power of this call to **choose.** And, in spite of my bruised sensibilities, and even my surprise at God's sternness, I knew in my heart that He was right. I could not continue to waver between two "realities." I had to choose whom I would follow. It was literally my life, now and forever. God was bringing me to this place of decision. That night, before I fell into my usual fitful sleep, **I think I finally did choose Him, with all the will I could manage.** And thus I began a new journey of preparation to see if He really would "answer by fire," although, as I just mentioned, I don't think that I really slept any better.

*(Note: I'm running my hand over the surface of my neck right now in that kind of absentminded, habitual, anticipatory way that I have done for the past eighteen months or so. Even this subtle, almost unnoticeable, but oft-repeated motion has been a journey unto itself.*

- *First, inquisitively, wondering about the mysterious lump,*
- *then, checking for its waxing or waning,*
- *then, kind of accepting its presence,*
- *then, being alarmed at the appearance of more lumps,*
- *then, fearful at the knowledge of the evil disease contained inside,*
- *then, with greater fear as the lumps seemed to grow even larger,*
- *then, with even greater fear and loathing as I imagined the incredible battle, both physical and spiritual, that was raging within them,*
- *then, with a troubled sense of surrender, faith, and apprehension as I realized my complete inability to control the lumps, or the disease, or the evil life which spawned it,*
- *and, finally, with caution and wonder, as I ponder what God has done, and what He may do next.*

*So here I am running my hand over the surface of my neck; I probably always will.)*

# CHAPTER 29

# (REALLY) LOOSE ENDS

As my radiation treatment progressed, the intense effect of the lethal beams was being branded, literally, into the skin on my face and neck. At first there was just the faintest outline of a mild "suntan" followed by an increasing redness. Then, the redness burst into full, raw bloom, which peaked for about a week after treatment ended. Over the next few weeks, the burns started to heal in reverse order, back to my now permanently tanned state. I remember being plagued by a nagging doubt about one small lymph node that was barely inside the treatment zone "boundary" that had been burned onto my neck. The lump was so barely inside the zone, that it might have been questionable whether or not it was receiving the full "benefit" of the "healing" rays. To this nagging doubt I added the fact that this lump had not seemed to change much, one way or the other. Thinking about this small lump represented yet another portal for the enemy's death whisperings to enter through. In my worst moments, I would imagine how a slight, human miscalculation in measurement and marking, causing this errant aim, might result in only ninety percent effectiveness, which meant leaving ten percent of the disease that was now possibly represented by the questionable, untouched lump, still positioned to murder me.

As I mentioned earlier, I would pray during each treatment session. I would pray for God to direct His healing will, both through clinical and supernatural means, toward **ALL** the cancer cells in my body, wherever they might be growing or lurking. Yet, it was evident that this nagging worry was another area of faith that needed to be addressed by Him. It's remarkable how my rough notes, recorded through this time period, indicate when these fear-to-faith issues had reached "critical mass." Even though the worries were more or less constant, I seemed to formally note the incidents when my heart was finally crying out to God. Many times throughout the journey, when I had reached this place of crying out, I would receive the answer through my now properly broken "heart of understanding." As for this question of whether or not the enemy was capable of somehow rendering treatment incomplete and perhaps only ninety percent effective, I had only to be reminded of the thousands of primary or recurrent cancer deaths to believe it possible, even probable. On the other hand, my own limited Bible memory recalled those scriptures which indicated that God was aware of **even a single sparrow's death, or that He knew the exact number of hairs on my head (Matthew 10:29-30).** This seemed to suggest that if God wanted cancer cells destroyed, He could easily destroy all of them. But, I needed something more substantial from Him; more current, more in keeping with the journey that I was on.

I managed to remember one more famous scripture passage about God's sovereignty. It was **Job, chapters 38 through 41,** where God answered Job's queries about Him from the midst of a storm. I turned to this passage and started to read. There were all of the Lord's thunderous words, affirming His power and His wisdom. And, in response, there were all of Job's words of understanding and inadequacy. The passage is generally considered to be very poetic and inspiring, and especially so, I thought, to a contented, healthy believer curled up beside the fireplace for his evening devotional, perhaps sipping a mug of hot chocolate. However, I have to admit that I was weary, tired, and ready to move on to another part of the Bible. Then, I read these words: **"Everything under heaven belongs to me" (Job 41:11).** My heart stirred with that familiar feeling of identity and recognition for words that I was supposed to read, and more importantly, hear. **That night, I wrote this brief entry in my notes: "God knows every detail – He will not overlook or miss anything – What the doctors may have missed, God cannot be deceived – He knows where every cancer cell is."**

It was strange how these words to Job, "from the midst of the storm," quietly ministered to me like **"a still, small voice" (1 Kings 19:12)** of assurance — a reminding voice. A voice reminding me that, yes, it was possible for inadvertent, clinical mistakes to be caused or even prompted by the enemy. But, even if human doctors had made a mistake, God's healing agenda didn't depend on the limited accuracy or effectiveness of the doctors or the treatment. He helped me see beyond the possibility that the enemy might have "sabotaged" my treatment, because the treatment itself was only a small part of God's healing resource. The treatments were just a minor "blip" on the radar screen that measured the "everything under heaven" that truly belonged to Him. Even if the enemy had arranged for some of the cancer cells to be untouched by human treatment, God's complete healing provision belonged to Him and only to Him. Those deviously hidden cancer cells would just be destroyed by another, unlimited Light Source. My peace with the future was slowly forming.

A few days later, I was busy reading one of my many "randomly" chosen books. It was a volume called *Journey*

*Into God* (**Augsburg Fortress, c. 2000**), dealing with the spiritual basis of healing in the temporal world. It was written by an internationally known speaker and Lutheran pastor, **Kenneth Bakken.** The book was very detailed, very scholarly, and quite a heavy read, but I had cultivated the habit of "hanging in there" with all the books I picked up. This perseverance was due to the many special, Spirit-led insights I had received during my free reading time. In order to properly set up this particular moment in my journey, I need to remind you of an entry that I had made in my rough notes, some **three months previous**, in the aftermath of my perspective-changing talk with Hope. It was during this talk that the image of the cancer idol first took tangible form. For your benefit, I'll repeat the entry:

**"The world bows to the idol of cancer...Doctors are the new oracles and high priests, and cancer clinics are the new temples...Is cancer the one disease where God does not have sovereignty?...Cancer makes us like new human sacrifices on the altar of human effort, knowledge, and treatment that secretly affirms death...Even the church has gradually been drawn in as a willing, but unwitting, participant in this mass delusion of the enemy....A great gig to get, if you're Satan...."**

As I worked my way through the book, I remember wondering if there would be any transcendent purpose realized, when quite abruptly, on **page 112** of the book, Bakken wrote these words: **"The high-tech, high-cost disease care system has, literally, become an idol. The hospital is the place of worship, and the medical specialists are the high priests."** It was time for me to be stunned again. Over three months after I had written my own words about the idol, I now discovered a parallel insight, written a couple of years previous, in a book that I had never read that was authored by a pastor who

I'd never met. My darkened mind reacted just a little, with prideful disappointment, that this principal "revelation" had not been "original" or given exclusively to me. (How difficult and embarassing it is for me to still confess selfishness and pride at this stage.) Then, recovering quickly by God's grace, I experienced the much more important reaction that I believe God had intended: encouragement. Reading this brief statement, in a single book chosen from amongst thousands of books, confirmed to me that it was truly an indication of **the Spirit of God being "poured out on all people" (Joel 2:28).** It confirmed that God was communicating with others about this issue as well. God was fulfilling my need for extra confirmation and encouragement to counterbalance the deeply embedded doubts and fears. Praise God for His faithfulness, again.

I know I said earlier that I wouldn't make you more weary of reading this account by endlessly rehashing stories of my physical symptoms or treatment side effects. But, I have been kind of waiting for a moment to tell you about some interesting "side effects of the side effects." These just seemed disturbing and weird at the time, but God would later use these experiences in a unique manner to validate Himself to me.

You will recall that the complete collapse of my taste buds, and my physical inability to eat real food, were the treatment side effects that were the most difficult for me to bear (even still, even with partial recovery of same). I confess that as the distance between me and the edible past widened, my longing, my discouragement, and my thoughts surrounding food became a constant source of torment, even an obsession, for me. To make matters even worse, a related side effect of treatment was an increased sensitivity to smells and odors. This sensitivity, when combined with my inability to eat, created vivid and frustrating "sensory food memories" for me on almost a daily basis. Nowhere was this "memory" more attuned than on my weekly trips to the supermarket, where I was determined to continue fulfilling my traditional duties of family grocery shopping.

I realize that you must think me a little masochistic to subject myself to an entire building complex devoted to foods that I could not eat or enjoy (maybe ever). I admit that for the first few weeks, it was difficult walking up and down each aisle, eyes playing over the shelves, remembering the aroma, flavor, and texture of all my favourite foods. It was especially difficult around the bakery and deli sections, where the actual smells of food were present and powerful. I do know why I stuck with this particular duty. I guess I wanted to be brave (if going to a supermarket could be called brave). I wanted to see if I could desensitize to my "addiction" over a period of time. As I have said before, I wondered if God was using this struggle as a method of uncovering yet another idol in my life (there were so many). As it turned out, I eventually was able to do grocery shopping in a kind of organized detachment. It was much like my "treatment bubble;" viewing the foods I placed in my grocery cart as just "packages of stuff" that other people ate. On the other hand, my "food memories" stayed just as acute as they ever were. In fact, I developed an even greater capacity to not only remember, but to imagine favorite food aromas and flavors. This would happen often, both voluntarily and involuntarily, and it became one of those classic love/hate relationships of my journey. *(Note: The **most** significant love/hate relationship was the wonder of experiencing God [the "love" part], through the "necessary" medium of cancer [the "hate" part]. I still can't honestly thank Him for cancer. I hope He understands.)*

I would find myself thinking about food almost constantly. Sometimes these thoughts were a good distraction from the fear and numbing reality that I was experiencing. At other times, they were a negative distraction, pushing me deeper into discouragement and envy, as I observed the "normal" reality of people living (and eating) all around me. And, I would dream; sometimes daydreams, and also night dreams. A couple of significant, food-related dreams stood out enough for me to make note of them (vivid and realistic like my business meeting, "CEO-asking-my-name" dream). I quietly suspected that these dreams about food had some transcendent meaning for my journey, and as God revealed other connections to me later on, this would, in fact, be true. Oh yes, and I think I noted them mainly because they were so bizarre, as well.

- The first dream didn't seem all that "real" to me, in the sense that I could tell immediately that I was in a kind of "altered" world. What seemed ultra real, however, was the unmistakable aroma of deep-fried chicken and french fries. I smelled this aroma as I, and a couple of unidentified "friends," crossed the street toward a small, fried chicken take-out place. I remember my mouth watering as we stepped through the doorway and up to the counter. I watched the attendant place the fry basket, filled with freshly breaded chicken, into the deep fryer. Suddenly, I was instantly transported and translated; **changed bodily into a fat, juicy drumstick, frying happily in the hot oil.** I remember sitting in the basket, looking down at my ever browning skin, as well as seeing my companion "parts" (breasts, thighs,wings etc.) cooking along with me. I wasn't being burned or harmed in any way, I was just able to experience the enticing smells and sounds of cooking in "first person" (or "first fowl"). The attendant took the basket out of the fryer and emptied "Fred the Drumstick" along with my succulent, golden brown companions, onto a serving platter. The aroma and anticipation of (someone's) first bite reached its peak, and then

I woke up. My mouth was actually watering (my salivary glands were still working at the time). As I sat there awake and somewhat in shock, I groaned quietly as I realized just how deeply affected I must have been by my extended, food exile. And yet, I was able to smile meekly as well, as I realized the sheer absurdity of being able to experience this dream as I did. **The next day I wrote this comment in my notes: "Last night, I dreamt that I WAS a piece of fried chicken…pathetic !"**

- The second dream occurred a couple of weeks later, I think, and this time it bore a greater resemblance to my business meeting dream in its sense of sheer physical reality. I was in a Denny's-like coffee shop, sitting around a familiar looking table with some unidentified friends. This particular setting resonated strongly with me, as I had shared many late night and early morning meals with my Convergence radio teammates at places just like this. It just felt true. I was also aware of being ill, and of being denied the pleasure of real food for a long time. For some reason, this occasion felt like my first serious attempt to eat real, solid food. The familiar noise and bustle of the coffee shop comforted and relaxed me, and I hardly noticed the plate of ham and eggs that the waitress placed in front of me. I remember thinking that I was approaching a moment of truth, of sorts, as I cut a small triangle of ham and placed a small morsel of fried egg on top of it, so I could eat them together. This was a natural, real-life habit of mine (another "normal" thing about the dream). As I placed the forkful of ham and egg in my mouth, I was overwhelmed with the discovery that the smell, taste, and texture were exactly, and perfectly, as I had expected them to be. And, as I chewed slowly, I became even more overwhelmed with emotion as I realized that for the first time in months, I was actually eating something real and recognizable. Just like a desert-thirsty man crawling to an oasis and drinking cool, spring water, I couldn't contain my feelings for even a second bite of food. I began to weep uncontrollably in gratitude, sorrow, and joy, right there at the table. I was so overcome by the grace of God, and by the taste of this incredible food, that I ended up sobbing face down on the table, head buried in my hands. Finally, after a few moments of this emotional display, I regained my composure sufficiently to look up at my friends sitting around the table with me. There they were; **Jerry Seinfeld, George Costanza, and Kramer**, all looking at me with a mixture of puzzlement and amusement. **I was a "character" in the TV show.** Jerry was about to make one of his patented, sarcastic comments about my outburst, when I realized that I was just in a dream, and I woke up. As discouraged as I was with all this, I remember laughing a little more about this one. It was still pretty pathetic.

A couple of days later, I told Warren about these dreams, as well as my mixed emotions of despair and quirky curiosity surrounding them. Warren ministered to me that day with a compassionate speculation about the dreams. Perhaps God wanted me to laugh with Him in the midst of a predicament that He fully intended to supernaturally resolve for me, albeit later on. This speculation, like other impressions that Warren had just "thought out loud" during our meetings, was to become much more prophetic weeks later. I didn't know this ahead of time, as usual, but I had to admit that even for me, there was a kind of deep and "dark" humor to these dreams.

# CHAPTER 30

# FIRST THINGS FIRST

It was now about a week before Phase I of my treatment evaluation; a follow up CT scan, plus an extra procedure called a PET scan (Positron Emission Tomography). The PET scan starts with an injection of a mild, radioactive solution into the bloodstream, which then gathers in areas of the body that exhibit unusual metabolic activity, such as tumor metabolism and reproduction. The PET scanning equipment then registers such areas, via the radioactive emissions, on a special photograph. It is considered an extra, double check on the limited accuracy of the other diagnostic protocols. I remember thinking that the prescription of this extra procedure was yet another move of God in my journey (I was told that not many patients were given such a scan).

The notion of the PET scan being a measurement of metabolic activity, both normal and abnormal, gave me a sense that God wanted to remind me what we were really dealing with. There was an "evil life force" which corrupted the normal functions of a human cell. In a way, the PET scan was a temporal tool that could partially detect the manifestation of this "evil life." This could have been just another musing of a man who was thinking about everything on a

24/7 basis. My thought life and my prayer life were focusing more and more on these critical few days ahead, which encompassed the two diagnostic scans and then culminated in the evaluation of the results. A follow-up consultation would complete the puzzle.

It had been four months since my first diagnosis, and my first, personal encounter with the demon. It had been four months of fear, darkness, light, struggle, and wonder. Now, the whole panorama of my experiences was narrowing down to this moment in time. It was like a magnifying glass, refracting and focusing the diffuse rays of the sun into a powerful pinpoint of light, centered on the truth. The deep, spiritual insights that I had been receiving, for months, all seemed to suggest (or declare) that I was moving toward a destination of healing, not destruction. And, beyond healing, there was a suggestion (or declaration) of new knowledge and purpose that would help others understand and receive healing as well.

So, I was praying everyday around this central idea of a "defining moment:" a moment when the "messages" of God received over the last four months would impact on the cold, temporal facts of the clinical assessment. I was actually petitioning God for a favorable outcome. I was asking for a clear indication that His "words" of healing, deliverance, insight, and purpose were, in fact, the Truth. I had "come out of the closet;" I was unashamedly asking God to "show me," like the Missouri state motto. I remember thinking that it was somewhat ironic that it would be the "priests of the idol," the doctors, who would in fact report to me on the validity of this "testimony."

As I recalled the story of Elijah's sacrifice to the Lord on Mount Carmel, I was struck again by his blunt call to decide between God and Baal. The story had taught me that the practice of believing in both gods simultaneously ("wavering" between the two) was just as destructive as the exclusive worship of an idol. **Elijah's challenge was consistent with what I had learned about the ongoing, mental debate between "reality" and faith. Intellectual stalemate was the same as defeat when looking for supernatural truth or healing.**

At the same time, when it came to cancer, the distinction between "reality" and faith was blurred somewhat by our acceptance of conventional treatment as a legitimate method for God to demonstrate His healing provision. It was clear that God had inspired mankind to discover and develop medicines and technologies to help cure disease. But, it was this very success that had led us to believe that we (mankind) were the "authors" of our own healing, the "masters" of our own destiny. Perhaps that was the reason God had allowed cancer to become such a unique and powerful destructive force. Perhaps God wanted to demonstrate that our forgetfulness of His authorship in the discovery of "man-made" cures was to make the cure itself, or man himself, the god. It was complex indeed, and probably one of the reasons why we don't see it with crystal clarity on our own. If we could see it with clarity, we might immediately act upon it by recognizing that the true foundation of all healing is God. As I reflected further on Elijah's story, I thought about his three-stage process.

- First, choosing to follow God exclusively;,
- and then, moving to a confrontation with the precepts and priests of the idol;
- and finally, with God's power behind him, confronting the idol itself.

**The story of the confrontation between Baal and God on Mount Carmel sets the stage to first test the faith and resolve of the chosen subject (victim or prophet), and then to demonstrate the power of the true God over the idol. I**

began to wonder if the picture of Elijah confronting the idol was a deliberate message to me. Could it be a message far beyond the call to simply choose "Who" I would believe? Then I remembered Gideon, the "mighty warrior."

I returned to **Judges 6–7** again, and re-read this first and favorite story that had been given to me. I was looking for the spiritual "connection" with the story of Elijah. As was the case with so many early readings, I was not to fully understand their significance until later on. At the appropriate moment, God would choose other texts or experiences to trigger deeper insights or clarify His meaning from those earlier readings. As I tackled the story of Gideon once again, I saw the familiar picture of the Midianite invasion being a "type" of cancer. Also, the account of Gideon's ordained mission to rid the land of the Midianite scourge provided me with renewed encouragement. But, there was something new, an anecdotal incident really, that stood out with a boldness that I hadn't perceived months before.

At that early stage, I hadn't really recognized the significance of the first words of Judges 6: **Again the Israelites did evil in the eyes of the Lord, and for seven years he gave them into the hands of the Midianites (Judges 6:1).** As you read further in chapter 6, it is clear that the "evil" spoken of was the practice of idol worship; specifically Baal and Asherah ("Aha!" exclaimed Sherlock Holmes). You'll have to take me at my word that, when I first read Judges 6-7 in October 2002, I was not really concentrating on the idolatry part very much. At that time, I was concentrating on the call of Gideon (especially because of the "mighty warrior" connection), the ensuing battle, and eventual victory over the Midianites. This early interpretation of the story gave me hope for a God-powered victory over cancer. Now, I had the Spirit-led understanding that idolatry was at the core of the demonic, cancer stronghold. And with the fresh insight provided by Elijah's story, I saw the importance and the supernatural timing involved in my return to the Gideon narrative. I know that I have remarked on how the scriptural imagery, throughout this experience, seemed to speak directly and very personally into my own circumstances. I have also remarked on how I had perceived something far more global, general, and even prophetic (there, I used "that word" again) in this same imagery. What I may not have remarked upon is **how this Gideon/Elijah connection seemed to transform the personalized aspects of the two stories into a kind of "instruction book" or "roadmap" for the events that I was now facing.** This "instructional" message was a new dimension for me to engage. It was even more amazing in its implications, but it also required even more faith. And for that reason, it made everything even more scary. Here's what I mean.

As I read, again, through the account of Gideon's call from God, I realized that the Midianites were not considered the "priority project" on God's agenda. **The idols, Baal and Asherah, were the priority.** It became clear that before Gideon was to embark on his fabled, oft-told journey of liberation for Israel, he **FIRST** had to complete a very important task for God. **Gideon had to tear down and destroy the altars of Baal and Asherah. Just like Elijah,** he was first instructed to participate in the confrontation with **idolatry, which was the central reason for Israel's suffering.** As I reflected upon this "first things first" theme in both stories, I was brought to a picture of my own impending meeting with the cancer idol: the diagnostic scans, and the follow up consultation with the doctors to discuss the results.

It was almost as if I was inside some kind of **"living parable,"** first threading its way through the Gideon and Elijah stories, and then repeating itself inside my own circumstances. I was overcome with the thought that, like Gideon and Elijah, God was somehow involving me in an eerily similar confrontation. I appeared to be approaching a confrontation with the priests of the idol (the doctors) at the "high place" of worship (the clinic). Most importantly, I was moving toward a confrontation with the power of the idol to dictate my future and eventually destroy me (the statistics, the limitations of treatment). In a way, I felt like I was actually being called to place myself into the spiritual "shoes" of Gideon or Elijah. By faith, I was somehow to transpose their spiritual confrontation with idolatry onto my clinical confrontation with cancer. God had been so faithful, over the last month, to demonstrate to me why this transposition was **real,** and now He was showing me, for the sake of my own life, why this transposition was **necessary.** Please don't think that I'm trying to place my own status with God alongside that of Gideon or Elijah. I'm merely saying that I believe God wanted to show me that **He wished to confront the cancer idol** just like He had confronted the idols of Baal and Asherah. The pictures of this eternal confrontation, timed by God to arrive at this critical moment in my own battle, encouraged me to petition and pray for the upcoming tests and results **to be the same kind of defining moment experienced by Gideon and Elijah.** This mysterious connection with the two biblical characters would continue and deepen as my "living parable" continued.

# CHAPTER 31

# PROMISES, PROMISES

Have you ever wondered what words or actions of God, in the Bible, constitute legitimate patterns of His "behavior" or "character" in our own, contemporary world? That's a silly question, right? But let's be honest: there isn't a believer who doesn't struggle with this question. We all struggle, with varying amounts of skepticism, with the assertion that God's Bible-recorded activity is both literal and demonstrable in our pragmatic, scientific world. As an example, we now know that naturally occurring, seismic or tidal activity can cause seas to "part," or that you can "raise the dead" with electrical stimulation of the heart, or even CPR. To avoid the struggle, many of us have concluded that it's far wiser to view the Bible in its allegorical or symbolic contexts as opposed to its historical or literal contexts. Once this logical step is taken, we create a "comfort zone" of co-existence (syncretism) between our sure knowledge of "reality" and the thematic "wisdom" of the Bible. In this way, we can see truth through a more complete, "modern" lens. We can avoid chasing after ancient, mythical fables that we think are just not reasonable for today.

I don't mean to open up an entire debate about whether or not this way of thinking represents the same kind of syncretism or convenient idolatry that the Bible describes. Nor am I in any position to say for sure what "truth" really looks like, other than what "truth" has come to look like for me as the Spirit has illuminated it. It is safe to say that when it comes to biblical concepts like healing, we all have a tendency to go to that comfort zone that I spoke of, especially when we are talking about cancer.

Being the typical, modern-day believers that we are, our sure knowledge of cancer's "reality" focuses us on the scientific treatments and statistics of cancer. On the other hand, our reluctance to completely reject the "wisdom" of the Bible causes us to interpret (or settle for) biblical terms such as "healing" to more accurately (and comfortably) describe "spiritual healing," leading to eternal life. This adjusted, right-sounding terminology enables us to avoid any kind of contradiction in our (un)comfortable sense of what's "real" or factual about cancer. In all fairness, so many people have died of cancer that no one could be blamed for wanting to stay in this "comfort zone." Had I not become ill, I would still be in that mindset myself. God had succeeded in jolting me out the "zone" and into a place where I had begun to see a new reality in His words and actions as portrayed in the Bible. These words were no longer just "wisdom" literature to be respected, discussed, and somehow patterned in our lives. These words were, instead, a true "reality" to be experienced and lived, not only *as if* they are real, but *because* they are real – and, because they are the truth.

As I approached the time of my own confrontation with the idol, I knew that, somehow, my commitment to this new reality was a crucial element in affirming the many experiences God had shared with me over the last months. The parallels between my personal situation and the biblical history I had "witnessed" were becoming unavoidable and intimate. The importance of my own commitment was only outweighed by the evidence of God's apparent, very personal commitment to me, through sharing the story with me in the first place.

It was almost as if He was promising me healing and victory if I could truly understand this new reality with my heart. It was **His** reality, lovingly and painstakingly communicated over the last four months. **This notion of having actually received a promise of healing from God** was a new threshold of faith that I wasn't sure how to cross. I wasn't even sure if I wanted to cross it, anyway. There were always new questions.

- Who was I to determine if God was promising anything (beyond what He promises any believer)?
- If God wasn't promising me hope and healing, according to the experiences and words I had been given, what was I supposed to be concluding?
- If I determined that there was a promise from God inside what had been communicated, how would I handle my total disillusionment if the promise wasn't fulfilled (which shouldn't be possible if it were from God).
- What if upcoming events demonstrated that I had not gotten it *all* wrong, but had just misinterpreted or misunderstood a crucial *part* of the message? Of course, this could still mean that I had misinterpreted EVERYTHING. My head was hurting just thinking about it.
- If there was no promise intended, was there *any* sure knowledge or wisdom that could be counted upon from all the experiences I had been given?
- Was any of it, in fact, real? My head was really hurting now.

As I pondered the last question, I realized that I simply could not "go there," because it *had* all been *so real*. I moved a step toward the threshold. Was the message not only a message of hope, but a promise, as well? There was barely any "comfort zone" left.

Have you ever read a book or seen a movie where the clues and evidence seemed to push you to some kind of "inescapable" conclusion? Remember when you were so sure of where the "facts" were pointing that it was difficult to get your mind off of the anticipated outcome? Remember the times when you missed just one, small piece of relevant information that rendered this "sure thing" completely wrong? In normal circumstances, one could appreciate these judgement errors as the result of clever writing or an elegant, literary misdirection that deflected and deceived. But, this potential for error became an object of great tension for me as I pondered the evidence of God's promises to me. It was yet another crisis of faith that God was leading me toward. The words, images, and experiences that I had received on the journey all seemed to point toward this seemingly inescapable conclusion of hope and healing. Yet, I was just human, and inescapably flawed in my thinking. I could be wrong, just slightly off base, but off base enough to render the act of turning these insights into "promises" a really foolish, even heretical, exercise. I mean, could you really "bind" God to anything? He was God, after all. At the same time, I realized that if I was slightly wrong in my interpretation of events, then everything was in question. And, if everything was in question, I could easily perish anyway in uncertainty, confusion, and fear. I couldn't believe that God would wish that kind of fate for me or for anyone else. So, I crossed the threshold with nothing to lose and everything to gain. I decided to explore my faith in His promise.

I had read a book on prayer, amongst other ongoing reads, which spoke of this concept of "binding" God to His own stated or demonstrated will. **The idea being that, if one was fortunate (or inspired) enough to discern God's will in a given situation, praying for the fulfillment of that will was merely affirming a foregone conclusion.** This was all based on the notion that God was infinitely true and dependable to follow through and deliver on His own stated intentions — His "promises," to put it another way. The apostle John gives the best description of this promised response.

**This is the confidence we have in approaching God: that if we ask anything <u>according to his will</u>, he hears us. And if we know that he hears us – whatever we ask – we know that we have what we asked of him (1 John 5:14-15).**

This kind of "praying according to God's will" is considered the ultimate in receiving sure responses to our prayers. How could one go wrong by praying for something that God already had ordained would happen? I'm not sure that I had ever been much good at discerning God's will in my former darkness of mind. I was content, like so many believers who think that they were living perfectly OK, normal lives, to keep that challenge in the "suspended" bin of the "God's Mysteries" section of my life library. Yet it appeared that God had decided to mercifully disregard my own discernment handicap in favor of a persistent, methodical, and "clear" expression of His intentions: by His Spirit and His Word. This book about prayer quoted a Scripture passage that verified God's desire to be infinitely true to us. The passage acted as an invitation, of sorts, to "bind" God to His own words and promises:

**<u>"Test me in this,"</u> says the Lord Almighty, "and see if I will not throw open the floodgates of heaven..." (Malachi 3:10).**

The implication of this text was that it was, indeed, OK to "test" God on what He had promised (not that He couldn't remember). It was like a child reminding his father of his promises to bring home ice cream for dinner, or to play catch in the backyard after chores were done. "Remember heavenly Father, you promised to do this. Now, will you?"

That same night, I began an open Bible reading of **Psalm 119;** a long read, as Psalms go. The reading began like so many had on the journey, with a kind of deep longing for God and a quiet regret that I had not been more transformed by His Word much earlier in my life. The first part of Psalm 119 reads like a combination lament, cry for help, bargaining session, and worshipful stream of consciousness. The opening verses are normal, fragile, fearful, and human. Then, as I reached verse 38, the tone changed, and the Spirit spoke again into my life, multiple times.

- **Fulfill your promise to your servant, so that you may be feared (Psalm 119:38).**
- **Remember your word to your servant, for you have given me hope (Psalm 119:49).**
- **My comfort in my suffering is this: Your promise preserves my life (Psalm 119:50).**
- **May your unfailing love be my comfort, according to your promise to your servant (Psalm 119:76).**
- **Sustain me according to your promise, and I will live; do not let my hopes be dashed (Psalm 119:116).**
- **Your promises have been thoroughly tested, and your servant loves them (Psalm 119:140).**
- **Defend my cause and redeem me; preserve my life according to your promise (Psalm 119:154).**
- **May my supplication come before you; deliver me according to your promise (Psalm 119:170).**

There was a reason why this psalm was so long. The psalmist had crossed the threshold ahead of me. The psalmist was being bold and persistent by challenging God to live up to promises that He had evidently given. Reading these very aggressive words to God helped me to see that it was not only OK to test Him in this manner, but doing so was, arguably, **an act of obedience in itself.** This important experience was designed to jolt me out of a standing position, to take me across the line to this new place of reminding God of His promises **to me.** I started praying the word "promise" the very next day.

# CHAPTER 32

# BIG THREE

The next few days of my life, just prior to my "final" diagnostic scans, were arguably the most significant moments of the whole, extraordinary journey. It was as if God had **"saved the best till now" (John 2:10).** I felt as if He wanted to encourage me for persevering with such a long, difficult story by giving me a brilliant and fulfilling solution to the current installment. I choose the term "installment" as though the story itself is going to be a continuing, extended volume about my life (the longer the better, I think). What I can also say is that, subsequent to the events I am about describe, God gave me a merciful, amazing, even sober sense of clarity about the unbelievable and seemingly unrealistic concepts that I had encountered over the last four months. These were spiritual concepts that I wasn't just observing or even just learning. I was actually **living inside** of these concepts, even as I lived out the temporal life that everyone else was watching. Praise God that I have the opportunity to allow you inside of these spiritual concepts as well.

The first moment occurred around 4:00 AM in another one of those quiet, solitary moments in my bedroom, while my family slept. I have already told you how these moments of reflection and prayer, in the aloneness of my soul, were among my richest and most encouraging moments in a perpetually difficult situation. Often, I had felt the presence of God around me as I sat in my sleeping chair, listening to the rhythmic breathing of my wife across the room. I would sit quietly, trying to peer into the darkness for some glimpse of God, straining my ears in the silence for some whisper from Him. On this particular night, however, my usual sense of quiet peace was replaced by something brand new. It was an "explosion" of a sort.

I had been dozing lightly, knowing that I would need to be awake in a couple of hours to take my son to school, when I was suddenly, and very abruptly, wide awake. Not just awake mind you, but consumed with an awareness of energy that was familiar in one way, but completely new and undeniably supernatural in another. We all can relate to those times when we were faced with a difficult problem of some kind, and then suddenly, almost spontaneously, we experienced a "Eureka!" moment. This is a moment when the problem and the solution merge into one amazing, self-evident picture. (Psychologists call this experience an "intuitive insight.") I had experienced my fair share of these moments throughout my life, and mostly, when I got past my own ego, I considered them a wonderful gift from God. For those more spiritually inclined, these moments of insight occur when one is faced with deep spiritual questions, problems, or puzzles that human logic just doesn't seem to address adequately. I experienced this kind of moment when the concept for our radio program, "Convergence Café," was born. It was a gift of creativity from God. (Believers often call this "divine inspiration.")

I can safely say that this particular moment for me, wide-awake and fully aware, dwarfed any previous experience, intellectual or spiritual (other than my first encounter with the Holy Spirit some fifteen years before). I just sat there in the dark, unable to concentrate on anything other than the overwhelming "waves" of knowledge that were sweeping through my mind and cascading over my heart. I realized that these waves were not of my own making. It wasn't like a dream, where you can rationalize that you provided the data for the dream from your own thoughts or desires. Nor was it like a regular idea or agenda, where your intellect or personality can be identified as the underlying foundation. This knowledge was spontaneous, unique, and more original than anything that I could have dreamt up on a moment's notice. It was both a snapshot and a movie. I knew that it had come to me from outside of myself because I could follow its individual steps as it unfolded, as well as see the whole journey as one complete map; both at the same time. It was like being directly plugged in to how God saw things. It was an amazing, enlightening story. **It was a story of how God actually cures cancer, completely.** Here's how it unfolded.

The first impression I noted was that the cure was only available because of **God's eternal nature**; that He doesn't exist in any normal sense of time. In addition, because cancer had been identified as a demon stronghold, a spiritual power underpinning the earthly disease, then the cure (by necessity) had to transcend time and temporal existence. Earthly medicine was not enough. God's eternal nature allows Him to exist and operate, simultaneously, in all the "zones" of time and space. God exists in both the physical and spiritual. He exists fully in the **past, present, and future.**

- **"I am the Alpha and the Omega," says the Lord God, "who is, and who was, and who is to come, the Almighty" (Revelation 1:8).**
- **With the Lord a day is like a thousand years, and a thousand years are like a day (2 Peter 3:8).**
- **Jesus Christ is the same yesterday and today and forever (Hebrews 13:8).**

I realized that all the teachings of the last few months, like the individual threads of the loom, were now being woven into that tapestry I had imagined, surrounding and adorning the Lord's very own nature. The healing "garment" was described to me like this:

- **"Past"...** Only God can identify, convict, heal, and cleanse the roots of hurt, pain, bitterness, anger, rebellion, and idolatry, which are **the roots that first create the conditions for the spirit of cancer to operate.** These roots need to be identified and healed in a kind of "retroactive" manner, as they were created sometimes far back into our past (possibly even originating in the womb or in previous generations). From such roots develop the wounds or openings for the demon to influence and infect us. God and the Holy Spirit have the power, and more importantly, the will to go back to the "beginning" of our wounding and repair our vulnerable spirit at its very foundation.

- **"Present"...** Jesus is alive, and the same today as yesterday. He can perform the same acts of healing and deliverance today that are described in the Gospels. It is no coincidence that most descriptions of His ministry intertwine the actions of binding and casting out evil spirits with the healing of the body. Jesus' combined ministry addresses **the two-fold nature of cancer: spirit and disease.** In this way, He binds and casts out the evil spirit of cancer and also enables healing of the physical manifestation of the disease. Another model of this kind of two-fold healing was illustrated when Jesus commanded the fig tree to die and it withered from the roots, underground, beneath human sight.

- **"Future"...** This part of the wisdom was the newest and the most amazing. It addressed the question that mystifies and frustrates clinical medicine. **Why does cancer often go into remission, then recur, and then kill? It is never really cured.** From the depths of my scripture memory, I was spontaneously given a paraphrase of the following text (the words of Jesus): **"When an evil spirit comes out of a man, it goes through arid places seeking rest and does not find it. Then it says, 'I will return to the house I left.' When it arrives, it finds the house swept clean and put in order. Then it goes and takes seven other spirits more wicked than itself, and they go in and live there. And the final condition of that man is worse than the first"** (Luke 11:24-26). Although I didn't recall this text in detail at that moment, I realized that I was being given **a spiritual picture of recurrent cancer.** The passage illustrated why cancer is rarely "cured" in the natural world. It was also a picture of how the enemy can use the delusion of "remission" to raise our hopes, and then afflict and torture us even more, later, when the cancer recurs. And then, our condition is literally "worse than the first." Somehow God was showing me that only He could fortify "our house" and indwell us with His life-giving presence, in order to prevent the future return of the evil spirit of cancer. It was a final, spiritual remedy that modern man could not understand. Only with this supernatural, "future treatment" could cancer be healed completely.

This whole experience seemed to take just a few moments that quiet night. It took much longer to write it down. I am still amazed. I'm also still wrestling with the question of how to seek and identify this "indwelling" that is part of our future victory over cancer. I am praying God will show me more clearly, so I can share it as well.

The next significant moment occurred a couple of days later during another open Bible reading session. I was paging through the New Testament this time, and found myself in the book of **1 Corinthians**. My eyes came to rest upon the heading **"Wisdom From the Spirit" (1 Corinthians 2:6)**. You know, I was never quite sure how God chose the timing to share scriptural insights with me. Somehow He always seemed to know the right moment to connect me to the next step, to reinforce and encourage me in what I had already seen. And, remarkably, He always chose the right moment to answer, specifically and directly, the many crucial questions that seemed to color so much of the experience. As with the answers to my questions about grace and election from Romans 9, it appeared that the apostle Paul was being used, again, to answer a question that had haunted me since the beginning of the journey. **How could I be sure that God was really communicating with me through this strange, new medium of scriptural pictures and images?**

I knew that John Sherrill's book (*He Still Speaks Today*) had gone a long way to illustrate a closely related kind of experience with Scripture, but so far I hadn't received anything "directly" confirming this unorthodox ("mystical," Warren had often called it) "play within a play" that I was "seeing" inside the actual words of the Bible. Besides, how was God supposed to do that anyway? It was difficult for me to imagine how God could confirm that the Bible was speaking directly to me **by speaking through the Bible**. For Him to provide this confirmation using the same mechanism (and source) of spontaneous, scriptural insight seemed to be the same thing as paying off an IOU with another IOU. The whole experience had taken on extraordinary, and yes, even mystical proportions. Events had gone way past the coincidental, or even the explainable-through-some-kind of-wishful-manipulation method. There was just no way that I was that creative or even that energetic to have deliberately fabricated so much of it. So, being completely aware of all this rationalization going on, God did not answer my question with yet another mystical experience. Instead, I began to read a very direct and clear "plain language" explanation of His mystical gift to me and how it worked.

- **We do, however, speak a message of wisdom among the mature, but not the wisdom of this age or of the rulers of this age, who are coming to nothing (1 Corinthians 2:6).** Now *this* made sense to me. The "wisdom of this age" (the cancer idol) urging the acceptance of "reality" certainly did not agree with the other wisdom I had been receiving. I wasn't so sure that I was very mature though.
- **No, we speak of God's secret wisdom, a wisdom that has been hidden and that God destined for our glory before time began (1 Corinthians 2:7).** The words "secret wisdom" echoed in my heart. I considered the possibility that what I had been "seeing" was the "wisdom that has been hidden" inside the words of Scripture. Was this hidden wisdom that had been "destined" for me?
- **None of the rulers of this age understood it, for if they had, they would not have crucified the Lord of glory…but God has revealed it to us by his Spirit. (1 Corinthians 2:8,10)** Just as in Paul's time, the "rulers" of my "age" (realists, doctors, skeptics, believers too) would have difficulty understanding and believing this hidden wisdom about cancer. But God was choosing to share it with me for His reasons and "by his Spirit."
- **The Spirit searches all things, even the deep things of God. For who among men knows the thoughts of a man except the man's spirit within him? In the same way no one knows the thoughts of God**

except the Spirit of God (1 Corinthians 2:10-11).
The "deep(est) things of God" were **His thoughts,**
and the Spirit knows those thoughts. The Scriptures
were not just arcane, written words on paper; they
were living, active thoughts.

- **We have not received the spirit of the world but
the Spirit who is from God, that we may understand what God has freely given us (1 Corinthians
2:12).** Some kind of connection has been made. We
have "received…the Spirit who is from God" so that
**WE** may understand just as the Spirit understands.

- **This is what we speak, not in words taught us by
human wisdom but in words taught by the Spirit,
expressing spiritual truths in spiritual words (1
Corinthians 2:13).** You could have knocked me
over with a feather. On one level, the printed words
of the Bible, the spoken words of friends, and the
written words of authors could all be engaged by our
human wisdom, subject to our human limitations.
But, the powerful, spontaneous images and insights
coming from deep within these human expressions
were being **"taught by the Spirit" to me.** They were
supernatural, "spiritual truths" in "spiritual words"
that I could only understand because of this special
action of the Holy Spirit.

- **The man without the Spirit does not accept the
things that come from the Spirit of God, for they
are foolishness to him, and he cannot understand
them, because they are spiritually discerned (1
Corinthians 2:14).** I knew that my story, if told to
the non-"spiritual," would sound like a fantastic piece
of desperate fiction from a desperate man facing a
desperate disease. Some of those people who loved
and respected my former, healthy persona might
"humor" me, sympathetically, but would not believe

me. Perhaps just a small remnant would *want* to believe me. Perhaps an even smaller remnant *would* believe.

- **"For who has known the mind of the Lord that he may instruct him?" But we have the mind of Christ (1 Corinthians 2:16).** Bring out the feather again. I know that there are some very learned, very serious explanations of this passage. **But, this was my immediate sense** about "who has known the mind of the Lord?" It was the Holy Spirit, of course. And the Spirit communicates the mind and thoughts of the Lord to us. In my case, the Spirit was communicating the thoughts of God to me through Scripture, the living Word of God. **So, it was not just the proverbial "living Word," but the actual "living" <u>words and thoughts of God</u>; the active "mind of the Lord."** The Bible was not just an historical, ancient, dead book of wisdom. By the Spirit, the Bible is one form of the actual living, eternal mind of God. And, in addition to the Spirit communicating God's mind and thoughts to us, **we have been given "the mind of Christ,"** which is the same thing as the mind of God. This communication (or connection) with God was more than just Spirit to spirit, or Heart to heart, but it was also **Mind to mind.** Amazing. Once the Spirit translates God's thoughts to the mind of Christ within us, it's no longer just some fantastic fable that has to be taken on faith. It represents the all-powerful, transcendent intellect of God. My scriptural story was not just supernatural and overwhelming in its temporal and eternal message. By the wisdom of the Spirit, the story was also intended to make **common sense** as well; at least for those who have "the mind of Christ" (God's "common sense.")

289

I still reflect on the power of this passage, even today. At the time, I just could not believe the clarity with which God had answered yet another of my core questions about the spiritual rollercoaster ride that I was on. I was not expected to merely interpret or even deduce a message inside some ancient, cryptic, biblical context. But in real time, **God was "thinking out loud."** God was sharing wisdom that only He could unveil, just as He had shared in Paul's time, or in Isaiah's time, or now, **in my time.**

The third installment in this amazing trio of experiences occurred just a couple of days before my final, evaluative scans. I had decided to try shoring up my faith a little, as the clock counted down, by re-reading some of the significant Scripture passages that had been given to me on the journey. I started at the beginning with **Isaiah 30:20-26**, which was **the very first passage** that I had noted in my makeshift "journal." This text had spoken of how my **"teachers will be hidden no more" (Isaiah 30:20),** presaging my providential encounter with the ministry of Dr. Sandra Kennedy. As I re-read the text once again, the **two other verses** that I had made note of, back in October, stood out yet again. At that time I wasn't sure of the precise significance of the verses, but they must have impressed me sufficiently to cause me to jot them down. But now, after so much more had happened, these innocent little notations took on a powerful, new meaning.

- **Whether you turn to the right or to the left, your ears will hear a voice behind you, saying, "This is the way; walk in it" (Isaiah 30:21).** I immediately thought of God's patient, relentless "shepherding" of my awareness over the last four months. My doubts and fears had often caused me to "turn to the right or to the left." God had faithfully prevented me from losing sight of His "way." Back in October, I had no idea what the "way" actually was.

- **Then you will defile your idols overlaid with silver and your images covered with gold; you will throw them away like a menstrual cloth and say to them, "Away with you!" (Isaiah 30:22)** This journey had become mostly about turning away from idolatry and then confronting it. These actions now involved my own personal idols, and of course, the cancer idol. Again, I was amazed **at what I now could see** about what I could not possibly have seen, back then.

I then read on to the completion of the passage that I had recorded in October up to **Isaiah 30:26.** As I read the final words of the verse, **"when the Lord binds up the bruises of his people and heals the wounds he inflicted,"** I remembered the feeling of hope that this passage had given me in the beginning. It was a message that God's hand was somehow involved in my affliction, and that He had a greater purpose intended for me. It was a loving purpose with a desire to heal, not to destroy. I remembered how important this belief had been throughout my struggle, especially with all the depth of sorrow, conviction, self-knowledge, and repentance that had taken place along with everything else. This belief in a greater purpose continues to be the singularly important motivation for me as I continue on this adventure. I came to the end of the original passage, but I felt an urging to read on into verse 27. As I read the first several words of **Isaiah 30:27, an image of the book of Nahum (my first insight into the cancer/Assyria connection)** suddenly entered my mind, and I knew that I had to continue.

- **See, the Name of the Lord comes from afar, with burning anger and dense clouds of smoke; his lips are full of wrath, and his tongue is a consuming fire (Isaiah 30:27).** Nahum begins with a similar expression of the Lord's "jealousy" (remember Hope's word from God?) and His "wrath" to be directed at the foe, Assyria.

- **His breath is like a rushing torrent, rising up to the neck (Isaiah 30:28).** Nahum's monumental declaration about how the Lord will **"make an end of Nineveh"** with **"an overwhelming flood" (Nahum 1:8)** resonated in my memory. This image of the "flood" was the very first "prophetic" statement that I had received about God's attitude toward the whole stronghold of cancer. This repeat reference to my ever-present, diseased "neck" just sealed the deal.

- **And you will sing as on the night you celebrate a holy festival (Isaiah 30:29).** Now that I believed I was supposed to read the rest of this passage, this reference to singing again, in celebration, encouraged my heart.

- **The Lord will cause men to hear his majestic voice and will make them see his arm coming down with raging anger and consuming fire (Isaiah 30:30).** Other people were going to witness His healing "anger," His majesty, and His sovereignty over cancer. I pondered the idea of my doctors, my family, my friends, and other cancer victims seeing God's healing arm coming down and being changed somehow.

- **The voice of the Lord will shatter Assyria; with his scepter he will strike them down (Isaiah 30:31).** There was that feather, knocking me over again. At the beginning, **I had no idea that this passage was about Assyria.** Here I was, four months after the original reading, being shown that the very first scripture I had been given was a well-hidden but very real description of the entire journey, even though I didn't know it at the time.

- **Every stroke the Lord lays on them with his punishing rod will be to the music of tambourines and harps, as he fights them in battle with the blows of his arm (Isaiah 30:32).** I read this part, now, with a renewed hope in God allowing me to worship and serve Him in music and song. Music would be an instrument of healing and victory in this prophetic war against cancer, and perhaps, against other idols.

- **Topheth has long been prepared; it has been made ready for the king [of Assyria]. Its fire pit has been made deep and wide, with an abundance of fire and wood; the breath of the Lord, like a stream of burning sulfur, sets it ablaze (Isaiah 30:33).** This was like a picture of Elijah on Mt. Carmel, confronting the priests of Baal. It was a picture complete with details about the "deep and wide" fire pit and the fiery "breath of the Lord." Topheth, like Mt. Carmel, was a "holy place" for idolatry (the worship of Molech) and human sacrifice in Isaiah's time. It was another image of the confrontation between God and the enemy.

OK, here's the thing about **Isaiah 30:20-33**: As I read the full length of it now with newly-opened eyes, it was as if God's mind was at work again. His mind communicated His faithful love, elegant intellect, and incredible, irresistible power. Back in October, God knew full well **that I would not have understood** much more of the passage than the first few verses. Yet, at the same time, He knew that I would come back to the text at this stage. God was now showing me something unique about His knowledge of the **"Beginning and the End" (Revelation 21:6)** and everything in between. This relatively short Scripture passage now read like a synopsis of my complete journey over the last four months. It was a little unnerving to consider that this **"treasure" had been "hidden in the field"** all along (Matthew 13:44).

Pardon me if I seem a little redundant, but this passage from Isaiah 30 was now like the "Coles Notes" version of the last four months.

- **Although the Lord gives you the bread of adversity and the water of affliction ... (Isaiah 30:20):** God's purposeful hand in my illness, complete with the Psalm 66 "prison" imagery (bread and water).
- **Your teachers will be hidden no more ... (Isaiah 30:20b):** Sandra Kennedy, Hope and Don, Warren, Lori, Laurie Lee, and oh yeah, the Spirit of God.
- **Whether you turn to the right or to the left...your ears will hear a voice..."This is the way" ... (Isaiah 30:21):** God's faithful, relentless, "multimedia"-style of communication and guidance on the journey.
- **Then you will defile your idols...throw them away...and say to them, "Away with you!" ... (Isaiah 30:22):** This journey was mostly about idolatry, and how idols separate us from the blessing of God. In addition to the cancer idol, I had noted eight other personal idols that God had uncovered inside my life.
- **...when the Lord binds up...and heals the wounds he inflicted ... (Isaiah 30:26):** This theme of God's ultimate, healing purpose still keeps me alive inside.
- **...with burning anger...his lips are full of wrath ... (Isaiah 30:27):** A reminder of Hope's original statements about God's jealousy over our surrender to the cancer idol, as also stated in Nahum.
- **His breath is like a rushing torrent, rising up to the neck ... (Isaiah 30:28):** Nahum referred to "an overwhelming flood" that would destroy Assyria. The "flood" would even reach up to my diseased neck. God had used this neck imagery to personalize the messages and comfort me throughout the journey. I

remembered John Sherrill's healing from head and neck cancer.

- **And you will sing as on the night you celebrate a holy festival ... (Isaiah 30:29):** I was reminded of His grace to me in preserving me from surgical mutilation. I was affirmed in my desire to worship Him, to sing for Him "in spirit and in truth" (John 4:23).

- **The Lord will cause men to hear his majestic voice and will make them see his arm coming down ... (Isaiah 30:30):** There had been some recognition, from close confidantes, that God's "voice" was speaking into my situation. We had all been praying for His purposes and His reality to be demonstrated more openly, more publicly. Perhaps this demonstration would take place during my upcoming examinations.

- **The voice of the Lord will shatter Assyria ... (Isaiah 30:31):** It was like God's "prophetic" promise to destroy my cancer and the entire, demonic cancer stronghold as well. (Spoken, just as Jesus had spoken to the fig tree.)

- **Every stroke the Lord lays on them...will be to the music of tambourines and harps ... (Isaiah 30:32):** God was addressing my discouragement over not having picked up my guitar or uttered a singing note for four months. It was a continued hope for one of my heart's deepest desires. Especially powerful was the depiction of **worship as a weapon** in the battle with the cancer idol.

- **Topheth has long been prepared...the breath of the Lord...sets it ablaze ... (Isaiah 30:33):** A confrontation was looming in the immediate future. It was a confrontation with the idol and its priesthood, represented by my scans, examinations, and consultations with the doctors. The passage ended with a picture of the eternal battle **beneath** the medical battle. It was a picture of victory and hope.

The events of the last few days had brought me to a kind of "ultimate moment" in my emotional and spiritual preparation for what was to come. I am still overwhelmed by the sense of timing and power that God displayed in sharing these three defining experiences, in as many days. He knew that I needed to be pushed over the edge, or at least **to the edge** of my faith. Yet, God still chose to be kind and patient. He knew that, in spite of the multiple experiences of the last four months, I still required Him to "write in big letters." As the morning of my scans arrived, I kept on praying. The picture of Elijah's confrontation with the idol was at the center of my spirit. **We would soon see if the cancer clinic would be my Mt. Carmel** (or just another "scientific" laboratory for naïve, reality-challenged, doomed rats.)

## CHAPTER 33

# THE TRUTH ACCORDING
# TO CAPONE

Leading up to the final examinations, my daily prayers
contained a fairly simple petition to punctuate the
lengthy list of "other stuff" that I always prayed for. I had
decided to depart from the characteristically complicated
way in which I normally attempted to understand, or even
just observe, most life situations. Instead, I would simply try
to "honor the vision" of my upcoming examinations being
like a modern day confrontation with the idol. And so, my
petition (paraphrased) went something like this:

**"Lord, in the name of Jesus, I believe that You have not
only shown me a vision of healing and purpose, but that
You have given me a <u>promise</u> of this healing and purpose,
inside Your Word, and in words to me. I believe that You
have also promised that cancer will not return to afflict me
again. I now humbly ask You to demonstrate this promise
in a way in which I will understand. I also ask that the
doctors will be puzzled, surprised, even perplexed at the
outcome of the tests. I ask that the results of the tests will
affirm Your promise of healing, and that I will require no**

**further treatment or surgery. I thank You for Your mercy and Your healing promise. In Jesus' name, Amen.**

My doctor had virtually warned me to prepare for less than 100% effectiveness from treatment, and to be "realistically" prepared for the possibility of radical neck surgery. So I reasoned that my own confrontation with the "oracles" who had predicted my future **hinged on my final belief in an outcome orchestrated either by the idol, or by God (a la Elijah).** My prayer reflected a commitment, or at least a turning, to the power of the true God over this idol. My petition represented a picture of how I hoped God would "answer by fire." I prayed this petition whenever I was thinking about the tests and slipping into fear, which was often. Yet in those final days before the scans, the sheer wonder of my long spiritual journey continued to comfort me, balance my spirit, and give me a sense of confidence as I moved toward the "showdown." The day finally arrived. One disturbing element of the last few days had been the realization that the swollen lymph nodes on my neck had not completely disappeared. They had certainly shrunk from the two months of treatment, but they were still there; much smaller, but still there. I must have felt my neck twenty or thirty (or much more) times a day, as if I could physically track their expected disappearance by examination time. But, they were still there as I entered the diagnostic imaging room for my CT scan. The scan took very little time, and as Lori and I waited for the film to be processed so that we could take it to the other clinic (where the PET scan was to take place the next day), I wondered. How was God going to deal with those infernal lymph nodes, which were obviously still there, and yet still carry through on His "promise"? I reverted to musing on how God had the supernatural power to change anything, including human cells and even photographic film in process. I don't think that I was any more afraid than I had ever been, but this "lumpy twist in the plot" added to the tension and drama of it all. I resisted the temptation to look at the developed films myself. What could I tell anyway?

The next day, we traveled to the other clinic to undergo the PET scan. You will recall that this is a special scan, requiring the intravenous injection of a radioactive liquid. The liquid "gathers" in specific, predictable locations of metabolic activity. It also registers the signature metabolic activity of cancerous tumors in other, unexpected locations. Although the CT scan only covered my head and neck regions, the PET scan was scheduled to map my entire upper body, which represented other potential areas for metastasis (spread). The interesting, and somewhat unnerving, aspect of this test was the notion that it was designed to detect metabolic activity; **a kind of "living disease" picture.** It fit in well with my view on the natural and spiritual "life" of cancer. The other clinic was different in design yet projected the same innocent, institutional image as the cancer clinic. And, it carried the same disarming spiritual atmosphere of processed death. The test took about two hours; the nodes on my neck hadn't disappeared since yesterday. I wondered how they would register on the PET scan. That night, I made two small entries in my notes; one for each of the last two days.

- **Tues, Feb 25/03…CT Scan – some small nodes left**
- **Wed, Feb 26/03…PET Scan – will there be any evil life anywhere?**

I had to wait another week to know the answer.

The next few days were kind of uneventful — painfully uneventful. I had plenty of time to ponder the journey, pray my prayers of petition, and of course, feel my neck. As far as the remaining lumps on my neck indicated, the "yoke" had not yet been taken from it. I thought a lot about the films taken from my CT and PET scans, sitting on some doctor's desk. I pondered the mystery of God's power, having the potential to alter the evidence on the film; paralleling the other unseen, supernatural changes inside my body. I thought about the incredible dilemma that God had placed in front of me. It was also a dilemma for those others (Lori, Hope, Don, Warren, Laurie Lee) who had closely followed my journey of new, spiritual insight. Just how "real" was all of this going to be? Beyond their love for me and the hope that burned in their hearts, I had (or God had) drawn them inside this drama that was now unfolding. For them, because they didn't have cancer, it wasn't necessarily a matter of temporal life and death, but it was, in a way, **a matter of life and death for their hope:** hope in a new, powerful horizon of Truth that God was evidently showing us all. Had I just made it "seem" so true, in the passion and wonder with which I had told them of each new insight? Was my passion and wonder merely fear and desperation in disguise? We had all been praying the same, specific, petitionary prayer regarding my test results. Had we been too specific, too narrow? Had we limited the healing vision of God by interpreting the journey in the way that we had done? It was starting to get too complicated again. It was easy to get mired in the many, seemingly contradictory "issues" of faith, such as:

- praying **according to** God's will vs. **for** God's will
- petitioning for "whatsoever **we** ask"
- the assurance of receiving, **if** faith is sufficient
- God's ultimate **sovereignty** to decide whatever **He** wishes
- the **real world evidence** of faith's failure
- the temptation to **rationalize the failure** so that God hadn't "failed"

My head was spinning, and weary.

The journey had been too real, too compelling, and too powerful to say that it hadn't happened, but it was still very possible to have missed a critical road sign along the way. It was possible to have taken a wrong turn, or fork in the road, which might lead to a mistaken faith destination, even though we thought that we were journeying toward the right place.

A number of years ago, the controversial, investigative television reporter, **Geraldo Rivera**, conceived and hosted a live, primetime, tabloid news event called (I think) **"Uncovering Al Capone's Secret Vaults."** It seems that, in the early 1980s, a routine engineering study of the legendary Lexington Hotel in Chicago (the prohibition-era headquarters of the infamous Mr. Capone) had uncovered a number of hidden, secret passageways and tunnels. These hidden tunnels led to remote locations throughout downtown Chicago, and were evidently intended to be used as escape routes, or, as passages for other clandestine movement. With the discovery of these hidden passages, other rumors (or legends) of secret hiding places, concealed inside the Lexington and constructed by Capone, started to circulate. These various rumors gave rise to a thin theory about a secret vault that Capone had constructed in the basement of the Lexington, to act as a depository for part of his vast fortune. The vault was believed to contain substantial amounts of illegal cash as well as jewelry and other interesting, valuable treasures stashed away by the mobster. A follow-up engineering study had revealed a hidden compartment in the basement of the hotel, concealed behind a massive concrete wall. It was there that Rivera brought the national television cameras.

For two hours, on live television, Rivera hosted, commentated, and spoke interesting bits of Capone history. He whipped up audience anticipation as the drills and hammers pounded down the thick wall which allegedly concealed Capone's "hidden treasure vault." I admit to being one of the millions of intrigued viewers who endured the painful two hours. We were all hoping — even believing — that we were going to actually see this modern day legend fulfilled. There were even some representatives of the U.S. Internal Revenue Service present, ready to officially document and take possession of the uncovered loot. Finally, as the last chunks of concrete were cleared away, I remember Rivera, utilizing his broadcaster's sales skills to raise our emotions to their highest pitch, saying something like, "The whole world is ready to see the secret of Al Capone's fabled vault!"

When the dust cleared and the lights illuminated the inside of the compartment, the cameras slowly panned over the buried treasure: **a few empty bottles and an old metal sign of some sort.** Even Geraldo seemed genuinely surprised and deflated by this unsatisfying conclusion. But, in true tabloid form, he tried to glaze over our disappointment and our anger at being misled. He spoke, in pompous tones, about the "fragility of legends," "the fine line between myth and reality," and "the continuing romance and mystery of Al Capone." He had succeeded in capturing our undivided attention, and secret hopes, for two hours, but nothing he could say would undo the fact that it had been a colossal waste of time. He had made his money and had taken advantage of our weakness and naivete. We walked away from our TV sets not only disappointed, but even more cynical than when we had started watching the program. We secretly wished that we had never started in the first place.

In my darkest moments of reflection, during these last few days preceding the discussion of my scan results, I wondered if my journey would end up like Geraldo's. The remarkable combination of longing and circumstance had birthed incredible expectations that could possibly end in the emptiness of broken dreams and an old sign that read "Wrong Turn." My own faith, and the faith of others, would not only be disappointed but would even diminish from the level it had been when we started the journey. It would be "one step forward, **ten** steps back." Cold reality would turn out to be what the world always said it was, and God would remain an utter, distant mystery.

In the midst of the stifling complexity that often occurred when I examined my experiences (which together were like a multi-sided, spiritual "Rubik's cube"), God mercifully intervened, again, but this time He did so to bring my thoughts and spirit back to a perspective of simplicity. He accomplished this through very simple and direct means.

My son, David, had been searching for a new job for about six weeks. He had read the newspaper classified ads each day, circling the prospects in red, and had dropped off literally dozens of applications. He had yet to be called for a single interview. I prayed daily for David in a general sense, but I hadn't directly petitioned God to help him in his job search; I'm not sure why. Two days before my consultation, I remember David feeling particularly discouraged about his long period of joblessness. For some reason, I decided to offer up a specific prayer to God, asking Him to provide an opportunity for David. **So, I just asked Him.**

Two hours later, David received his very first phone call requesting him to attend an interview the next day. I remember feeling at first a little shocked, and then encouraged, and then finally aware of the message in my spirit. I felt God was trying to tell me that He could answer prayer simply and directly. God was also telling me that He could answer **my prayer** simply and directly. If God cared about something as "small" as a part-time job for my son, how much more would He care about the prayers regarding the future of my life, both now and in eternity (sounds like Scripture...hmmm). I don't think that I had often experienced this simple kind of answer to my prayers, at least at a time when I so needed to know if He would answer. Again, I praise God for His timing.

# CHAPTER 34

# THE KING OF CANCER

The next day, now just twenty-four hours prior to my consultation, I was trying to do some more open Bible reading. I was paging through Isaiah, again, more or less convinced that I had received, from this incredible book, most of the knowledge that was destined for me. I reached **Isaiah 13** and saw the heading **"A Prophecy Against Babylon."** For some "unknown" reason, I glanced at the footnote reference for this chapter in the bottom margin of the page. The footnote stated that the name "Babylon" was referring to this region during the time of the Assyrian dynasty. The boastful Assyrian kings often liked to award themselves multiple titles, such as "King of Babylon," to accentuate their own greatness. **This prophecy was actually against Assyria,** my picture of the cancer stronghold. I began to read with new interest.

Isaiah 13 unfolded with a repeat picture of the cruelty and arrogance of the Assyrian monster. There were even more vivid descriptions of God's anger and His intended destruction of the insolent, ruthless conqueror. This was encouraging, but without new insight. I continued the reading of the prophecy through Isaiah 14 with similar results, and was now thinking that this quick scanning would be over soon.

Then as I reached **Isaiah 14:12**, my heart jumped as I read these words:

**How you have fallen from heaven, O morning star, son of the dawn! You have been cast down to earth, you who once laid low the nations! You said in your heart, "I will ascend to heaven; I will raise my throne above the stars of God; I will sit enthroned on the mount of assembly, on the utmost heights of the sacred mountain. I will ascend above the tops of the clouds; I will make myself like the Most High (Isaiah 14:12-14).**

I was very quiet for a moment. I realized that I was reading **THE** Bible passage that was generally recognized as the definitive text for the entire, monumental battle for eternity: **the casting out of Lucifer from heaven.** I didn't know what to say. I was familiar, in a paraphrase manner, with this text, but I didn't expect to find it here. Yet, I was sensing, with some clarity, why I was reading it now, and reading it here, inside this prophecy against Assyria, my cancer foe. I believe that God was telling me one more important, faith building "fact" about this journey. He was encouraging my heart to believe Him as I prepared to enter the tabernacle of the idol. **God was telling me that the connection between Assyria and Lucifer was not coincidental.** He was telling me:

- That just as the story of Lucifer was scripturally intertwined with Isaiah's prophecy against Assyria, so was Lucifer spiritually intertwined with the demonic stronghold of cancer.
- That the force behind cancer was not just demonic, but **Satanic.**
- That amongst many of the diseases in the world, cancer was distinctive, because **the enemy himself was at the very center of its power.** In a resonant

way, this significant text about Lucifer was at the center of the prophecy against Babylon (Assyria).

- That even if Satan was not the substance of the stronghold, he was, at least, the **evil "heart"** of the stronghold.
- That I was not imagining anything. That I could believe God for the knowledge of the evil stronghold that He had shared with me over the last months.
- That there was a supernatural, and wholly reasonable, "logic" to the story that God had chosen to unfold for me.
- That I was not crazy.
- That I was loved, and had been entrusted with His deeper wisdom.

My heart was fuller than it had ever been, which was a good thing, since tomorrow we would face this same enemy, this same demon, this same idol.

# CHAPTER 35

# CONVERSATION ON MT. CARMEL

The morning of the examination arrived, and as best as I could, I prayed my petition to God. I added a message of surrender and trust along the lines of **"Into Your hands I commit my future."** It was difficult to be that brave, but I said the words anyway. Lori and I arrived at the clinic a little early, and as we sat in the waiting area, I realized that it had been a month since I had last ventured into the "lair of the lion." I hadn't forgotten anything, but I was reminded of the power lurking there as I watched my fellow victims. Some of them were obviously there for their first visit, hovering between hope and hopelessness. (O God, may Your Word be true.) I think Lori and I were both praying silently as we waited to be called. I felt my neck for the umpteenth time; yes, the little lumps were still there.

Finally, my name was called and we were led into one of the small examination rooms. While we were waiting there, Lori had to go to the washroom, and just after she left the room, the door opened again, and my radiation doctor poked his head inside. He asked where Lori was. I told him, which caused him to say that he wanted to wait for her return before the consultation started. I immediately thought, "OK, the enemy is throwing one last stress bomb into this situation, making me wait just a little longer." The doctor was drawing his head back out into the corridor, when it was almost as if he sensed that my silence, deafening as it was, was worthy of a second thought. He popped his head back in and said, **"By the way, both scans came back <u>clear</u>.** We'll talk more when your wife returns." The door closed again.

I sat there for a moment, lost in a disbelieving kind of "otherness." I wasn't really lighthearted or particularly heavy-laden. I wasn't really afraid, but I didn't feel courageous either. It was like receiving a package from your enemy and expecting a bomb, but getting home-baked muffins instead. Then, wondering if the muffins had poison inside them, just after taking a first, hungry bite. I had heard him say it: "clear." Yet, the fingers on my hand automatically went to the spot on my neck where the remaining small lumps were still palpable. It seemed like a long time before both Lori and the doctor were back in the room with me, and though I had enough time to say the word "clear" to Lori, we both listened intently as the doctor explained just what he meant.

> "Both the CT scan and PET scan have come back "normal," Mr. Tamagi, which means that we can't see any cancer in those areas where we originally targeted, nor anything suspicious in those other areas, like your chest, where we might expect it to spread."

> "What about the small lumps that I can still feel on my neck? Did they not show up on either scan?" I asked right away.

> "Let me check again." He read the reports over again. "No, the CT scan reports no physical detection of them,

and the PET scan doesn't mention any metabolic activity in your neck."

The doctor examined my neck, and after some probing, acknowledged that he, too, felt some small, leftover nodes. "Keep in mind that the CT scan may not pick up masses below a certain minimum size, and we tend not to worry about them if they are that small. But you do, certainly, still have some small nodes there, even though I had to work a bit to find them." (*You just haven't felt them as often as I have*, I thought.)

"I should mention that the PET scan works the same way," the doctor continued. "Below a certain threshold the scan will not pick up any activity, so there could be minute amounts of cancer still present, but not enough to cause the radioactive material to gather and register." (The idol was already demanding to be acknowledged, I thought.) "However, the PET scan is still really helpful, in a general way, to support the data from the CT scan. It all looks pretty good, for now." *For now.*

"What about these nodes?" I asked.

"Well, for now I think that we should just watch them to see if they stay the same, or even continue to shrink, and then disappear."

"Then, you don't think I need neck surgery right now?" I was thinking about our prayer of petition.

"I don't think that we need to jump into that right now, no. But your surgeon is in the clinic today, and I'd like him to come in and talk to you a bit before we decide completely." (*Uh oh.*)

The surgeon entered the room and quickly flipped through the scan results. He looked at the radiation doctor and said, "You did good." Then he looked at me, and he spoke.

"In a situation like this, it's really a personal decision whether or not to go ahead with a neck dissection, even with pretty normal results like these. Because, in spite of what the scans tell us, they are still limited, and the only way that we can be completely sure if there is any cancer activity or not is to take those nodes out surgically and look at them under a microscope. But, in your case, we don't have to do that right away. We could wait and see."

"You mean that you're not recommending or urging me to have the surgery, right now, just to be sure?" I asked pointedly.

"No, I'm not insisting," the surgeon replied. "But I can tell you that it would be a lot easier to do it now rather than later. The radiation has a progressive effect on the tissue and muscle that's been treated. As time goes by, it gets tougher and tougher to cut through properly and do a smooth surgery in that area. **I just did a neck dissection on a patient who had a similar cancer TEN YEARS AGO.** It wasn't very pretty (*Why did he say that?*). So if you're asking me if I'd rather do surgery now as opposed to a year or two from now, I'd say now."

I decided to extend the discussion. "Well, I still have these small nodes on my neck, but they didn't register on either scan for some reason." I wasn't sure if I was helping my case or not. The surgeon examined my neck for a while.

"I can't really feel anything," he remarked, and shrugged his shoulders. (*You **can't** feel them, I **can** feel them, the radiation doctor **can** feel them; ARE THEY THERE OR NOT?!?" I thought loudly.*)

"So, if I had the neck surgery, just in case there is some undetectable cancer left in my lymph nodes, I guess that will improve my chances of survival?" I was "cutting cards with the devil" a bit, as if my chances of survival were really in the idol's hands anyway.

"Oh no, it won't really change your chances of survival, but it will improve local control of the disease. Surgery can help prevent reoccurrence in your neck area, but overall, the survival rates for your kind of cancer haven't really changed in forty years," replied the surgeon matter-of-factly.

"You're saying that if I have surgery, my chances of survival don't really change, but 'local control' means the chance of reoccurrence in my neck is reduced. Why should I have surgery then?" My head was starting to spin again.

"Hey, don't knock the benefit of local control," the surgeon replied. "This guy that I just operated on had his first neck cancer ten years ago, and like I told you, this surgery was not easy, and was much more difficult all around." He was getting a little irritated with me. "But, either way, there's no sure way of knowing. We could do the surgery and find nothing, or be very glad we did do it, because the scans possibly didn't detect everything."

Radiation doctor added his voice. "Yes, that's true, 'local control' is a very important factor in the patient's quality of life in managing the disease. But it's possible that those small nodes are just scar tissue, or it's even possible that they were just reacting, normally, to the cancer further upstream, and perhaps never, in the first place, contained cancer cells themselves. We just can't know for sure without surgery. But it's not an obvious situation for surgery, either. I think what we are saying is that you **could** have surgery. It might even be prudent to do it, while you are younger and stronger. But we are not pushing you to have it. We could just monitor you closely and wait and see. I actually think that's what we should do." The surgeon agreed with the idea of monitoring, but I had the feeling that he was thinking, "sooner or later..." He left, kind of abruptly.

I couldn't resist the temptation to ask the radiation doctor, "Are you kind of surprised at the outcome of the treatment? You seemed cautious at the end of January, as if trying to prepare me for the likely possibility of surgery. Are you surprised?"

He replied, "Yes, and no. Yes, because at the end of treatment, the lumps didn't seem to be shrinking as fast as I'd hoped, even though they weren't that big to begin with. And No, because it proves that every cancer can respond differently to treatment, and there's a lot of the outcome that we just can't control or know for certain. There's a lot we just don't know." (Later on, remembering that comment, I wrote in my notes, "The doctors know that they fight a beast!")

He continued, "I think that we should just do another CT scan in a month's time, and if that's clear, then we'll just watch you closely. In the meantime, congratulations.

Why don't I let you and your wife go home. I'm really pleased, Mr. Tamagi."

Lori and I left the clinic. I would return for another follow-up CT scan in a month's time. We were grateful, quiet, relieved, numb, and feeling the mystery of God, deep inside the layers of this experience. I wondered if the radiation doctor felt the mystery, as well, and just could not "realistically" admit to it, even if he was a little surprised at the outcome.

# CHAPTER 36

# SPIRITUAL PALINDROME

I decided to write the previous chapter in a slightly new way, in a "conversation transcript" form, for a reason. And, I only came to understand the reason for this approach during the actual writing. It's almost as if I had to formally re-write my memories, now, of that incredible exchange, to view it with the same intense, yet dream-like attitude that had colored the actual experience then. It's also because of the "delayed reaction" insight that I received in the hours and days following.

It was almost as if the consultation had played out just like the Biblical narratives that God had used so powerfully in the preceding months. The experience became yet another medium to let me see my story inside His story. As I view it now, this truly was a new experience for me. **Instead of speaking to me first from the spiritual realm via Scripture, dream, or book, and then connecting this new "reality" with a temporal experience, God was reversing the process.** It was like a magician who shows the audience both sides of the curtain before he makes something appear or disappear, or an engineer who throws a machine in full reverse mode to demonstrate that it works equally well, forward or backward. *(Note: For the uninitiated, a "palindrome" is a word or phrase* *that reads the same forward or backward. Examples would be the word "deified" or the phrase "Cain, a maniac.")* With this real-life "Bible narrative" taken from temporal events in the clinic, God planned for me to connect the words and actions of its real human characters to new insights in the spiritual realm. Perhaps He wanted to know if **I** would "work" equally well, forward or backward. What were the connections between this "live report from the front lines" and His incredible, transcendent, healing truth?

The first, humbling, amazed thought that I had, as we drove away from the clinic, was the fact that my prayer of petition, repeated so many times prior to this day, **had been, quite simply, answered in detail.**

- I had prayed for a healing to take place in a way that I would understand. The scans had been clear, the report had said "normal" (for now). Pretty simple, straightforward, easy to understand.
- I had prayed for surgery not to be necessary. Somewhat begrudgingly on the part of the surgeon, surgery had not been prescribed or even recommended (for now).
- I had prayed for further treatment to be unnecessary. I was just going to be "monitored" (for now).
- I had prayed for the doctors to be puzzled, surprised, even perplexed by the outcome of my treatment. Both doctors had either admitted or displayed some surprise and perplexity at the outcome.

  - There had been the expectation for surgery that was now unnecessary.
  - There was the fact that my remaining, small nodes did not appear on either scan.
  - There was the surgeon's inability to detect the same nodes that I, and the other doctor, still felt on my neck.

- There was the surgeon's thinly veiled irritation at not "getting the surgery over with."

Regardless of the ever-present, spoken qualification "for now," I couldn't escape the wonder, awe, and fear around the fact that God had answered my prayer, in a sense, "to the letter." This was decidedly not like praying for my son to get a job interview.

The second connection occurred a little later that same day as I continued to ponder the strange contradiction of the remaining small lumps. I could still feel them on my neck, and I continued to be intrigued by the fact that they had failed to show up at all on either scan. These residual lumps had even been a subject of mild debate under direct examination by two doctors. Quite abruptly, my mind was taken back to a scripture passage that I had read back in mid-December, over a month prior: **Isaiah 10:5-27.** Although other parts of this scripture had been made clear during the course of the journey, **verses 16-19** had puzzled me then, but now they suddenly became like the spiritual "echo" of the most recent events at the clinic.

**Therefore, the Lord, the Lord Almighty, will send a wasting disease upon his sturdy warriors; under his pomp a fire will be kindled like a blazing flame. The Light of Israel will become a fire, their Holy One a flame; in a single day it will burn and consume his thorns and his briers. The splendor of his forests and fertile fields it will completely destroy, as when a sick man wastes away. And the remaining trees of his forests will be so few that a child could write them down." (Isaiah 10:16-19).**

I had seen and learned so much over the last few months.

- The picture of Assyria as the cancer stronghold.
- The images of fire raining down from heaven to consume God's enemies in Isaiah's time and in Elijah's time.
- The connection of this healing fire to the "forests" and "trees" of the enemy (the cursed fig tree of Jesus and the doomed "fig tree" fortresses of Nahum's prophecy). These "trees" and "forests" were pictures of the disease itself.

Yet, I had been puzzled by the seeming **contradiction** of the last three lines in this scripture. **First, there was the promise to "completely destroy" the "forests" of the enemy, and then, the competing reference to "remaining trees."** I had wondered how God could heal a disease "completely," and yet leave some disease behind, or "remaining," if my spiritual sense of this scripture was correct. Now, six weeks later, I think I finally understood. God had become a healing fire, and He had "destroyed the forests of the enemy;" the scan results had detected no "evil life." Right up until this moment, there were still some small nodes left on my neck; reminders of the disease. These nodes could not be seen on the scans nor even detected consistently by human touch. **They were, in fact, "the remaining trees,"** even as the "forest" had been destroyed. And yet, the "remaining trees" were "so few" (and so small) that sophisticated medical machinery could not "count them," nor could one of the doctors actually feel them. (Naturally it was the surgeon who appeared to hold on to "reality" with the coldness of surgical steel.)

Yet, **I could still feel the lumps**. I had this picture of a small child, innocently running his hand over my neck, and saying that there were some "bumps under there." It was an image of a true child, unspoiled and unencumbered by the crushing weight of scientific realism. **Or, was I the child, still growing in faith?** A child simple enough to count the small things, simple enough to believe the unbelievable, simple enough not to bow to "reality"? I felt like a child, to be sure, yet not the kind of child that the Bible speaks of. I was not the kind of child that simply trusts the Father with everything. Most of the time I just felt immature and weak.

There was, however, a deep, compassionate message in this re-acquaintance with Isaiah 10. Now, by identifying the reference to "the remaining trees," God was telling me, again, that this experience was real. He was, by grace, allowing me to see my life inside the living words of His Mind: His Scripture. God had chosen Isaiah, thousands of years ago, to write the words "remaining trees." He had now chosen this moment to unlock the "hidden wisdom" inside Isaiah's ancient words to describe His mighty works inside my life.

The lumps have since disappeared (**"as when a sick man wastes away…"**), but I think I'm still counting them.

# CHAPTER 37

# JUST A BATTLE, NOT THE WAR

Over the next few days, I continued to recover from my confrontation with the idol. I reflected upon the months of treatment, struggle, prayer, and of course, God's wondrous journey. I felt spent and a little "shell shocked." It was a strange condition for someone who, from now on, **will never actually leave the battlefield.** Cancer "healing" is like a battle that must be won, and won again, day after day, grace after grace. I was, also, still battling the enemy in my mind. The whole vocabulary of cancer's uncertainty had been launched at this "child" who was still counting the trees.

- "You're fine, for now."
- "No surgery, for now."
- "There could still be cancer activity, just below the detection threshold; we'll just have to wait and see."
- "Oh, the survival rate for your cancer hasn't changed in forty years."
- "I just operated on a guy who had a recurrent cancer **TEN YEARS after** his first episode."

After the initial "euphoria" (there must be a better word) over the "normal" test results, it was as if the doctors had spent the rest of the consultation preparing me again for the worst. It was as if they were telling me not to get my hopes up too high or believe in too much of a future. It was like they couldn't help but believe, with all their experience, that the future held anything other than death. The "monster" occasionally got beaten back or went into hibernation, but it didn't ever really go away. I admit to still being haunted by these words of discouragement, and yet, God faithfully leads me back to His reality, so painstakingly constructed in my heart over the months. A couple of days after the consultation, He demonstrated one more time that I was deep inside His eternal story. My heart was again encouraged to hope in Him, and to believe in a purpose that was still possible for me.

Call it another inspiration from God, because **I began to see another strange pattern** in the way the doctors responded, with almost spontaneous qualifications, to any notion of complete victory over the disease. It was a cautious "realism," preparing for the worst. As I said right at the outset of this now very long story, I could see why they did this in the name of compassion, having seen so many occasions of dashed hopes and eventual failure. The "strange pattern" I noticed had more to do with the sequence of events inside the consultation, representing the "confrontation with the idol" itself. **Something about this pattern caused me to look once again at the biblical descriptions of Gideon's and Elijah's confrontations with the priests of Baal.** I wondered if there would be another marvelous connection. I wasn't disappointed. There was yet one more chapter to my story that God wanted to unveil through these passages.

- **That same night, the Lord said to him (Gideon), "…Tear down your father's altar to Baal and cut down the Asherah pole beside it. Then build a**

**proper kind of altar to the Lord your God ...So Gideon took ten of his servants and did as the Lord told him ... In the morning when the men of the town got up, there was Baal's altar, demolished, with the Asherah pole beside it cut down ... They asked each other, "Who did this?" When they carefully investigated, they were told, "Gideon, son of Joash" did it. The men of the town demanded of Joash, "Bring out your son. He must die, because he has broken down Baal's altar and cut down the Asherah pole beside it" (Judges 6:25-30).**

- **Now Ahab told Jezebel everything Elijah had done [Baal's altar had been destroyed on Mount Carmel] and how he had killed all the prophets with the sword. So Jezebel sent a messenger to Elijah to say, "May the gods deal with me, be it ever so severely, if by this time tomorrow I do not make your life like that of one them."(1 Kings 19:1-2)**

I was amazed again. It was like the picture of my own confrontation with the cancer idol. First, the "destruction of the altar" (no human sacrifice allowed, this time) via the normal test results, and then, the almost automatic qualifications about future defeat and possible death. The "compassionate realism" pronounced by the doctors on the heels of my "good results" had supernaturally merged into these scenes from the lives of Gideon and Elijah.

All three of us had been led to the confrontation, all three of us had witnessed the grace and power of God, and **all three of us had received immediate threats of death.** It was like God was saying to me, again, that my life was inside this same eternal battle, alongside of these amazing men of purpose. (I am still hesitant to write this. I am no Gideon. I am no Elijah. I am still trying to figure this out.)

Gideon and Elijah had both received serious death threats, but neither one died as a result of these threats. This was because the threats were uttered by followers of a defeated idol (and in my case, involuntary, unsuspecting "followers"), and **because God had plans of additional purpose for both of them.** I sat back in wonder, anticipation, and tension as I thanked God for showing me another spiritual connection with these men of God. I wondered, humbly and fearfully, how far He planned to let the connection evolve. For with purpose there was also a future.

I now stand healed, today. I will wait for news of this same healing as I awaken tomorrow, by the grace of God. I will wait each day for His grace, as I wait, also, for my purpose and my future. I sense that my healing will go on for as long as my purpose goes on. Only my Counselor knows what my purpose is. I trust that He will instruct me, as He has so faithfully done these last months. If my purpose is to be realized in the fullness of time, only my Healer knows how long that will be. But for now, I stand healed, amazed, irradiated…illuminated. Amen.

Printed in the United States
47114LVS00002B/49-108

9 781597 818469